ACTION PLAN FOR

HIGH
CHOLESTEROL

J. LARRY DURSTINE, PhD

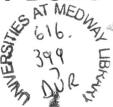

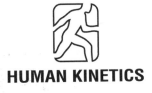

HUMAN KINETICS

Library of Congress Cataloging-in-Publication Data

Durstine, J. Larry.
 Action plan for high cholesterol / J. Larry Durstine.
  p. cm.
 Includes bibliographical references and index.
 ISBN 0-7360-5440-5 (soft cover)
 1. Hypercholesteremia--Popular works. 2. Blood cholesterol--Popular works. I. Title.
 RC632.H83D87 2006
 616.3'997--dc22

                                    2005017332
 ISBN: 0-7360-5440-5

Acquisitions Editor: Martin Barnard; **Developmental Editor:** Leigh Keylock; **Copyeditor:** Alisha Jeddeloh; **Proofreader:** Erin T. Cler; **Indexer:** Betty Frizzéll; **Permission Manager:** Carly Breeding; **Graphic Designer:** Fred Starbird; **Graphic Artist:** Francine Hamerski; **Photo Manager:** Dan Wendt; **Cover Designer:** Jack W. Davis; **Photographer (interior):** Dan Wendt, unless otherwise noted; **Art Manager:** Kareema McLendon-Foster; **Illustrators:** Figure 2.1 © Human Kinetics; figure 2.2 © P. Dennis/Custom Medical Stock Photo; figures 2.3, 3.1-3.3, and 4.1 by Kareema McLendon-Foster; **Printer:** United Graphics

ACSM Publication Committee Chair: Jeffrey L. Roitman, EdD, FACSM; **ACSM Communications and Public Information Committee Chair:** Harold W. Kohl, PhD, FACSM; **ACSM Group Publisher:** D. Mark Robertson; **ACSM Editorial Manager:** Lori A. Tish

We thank Body Tech in St. Joseph, Illinois, for assistance in providing the location for the photo shoot for this book.

Human Kinetics books are available at special discounts for bulk purchase. Special editions or book excerpts can also be created to specification. For details, contact the Special Sales Manager at Human Kinetics.

Printed in the United States of America   10 9 8 7 6 5 4 3 2 1

Human Kinetics
Web site: www.HumanKinetics.com

United States: Human Kinetics
P.O. Box 5076
Champaign, IL 61825-5076
800-747-4457
e-mail: humank@hkusa.com

Canada: Human Kinetics
475 Devonshire Road Unit 100
Windsor, ON N8Y 2L5
800-465-7301 (in Canada only)
e-mail: orders@hkcanada.com

Europe: Human Kinetics
107 Bradford Road
Stanningley
Leeds LS28 6AT, United Kingdom
+44 (0) 113 255 5665
e-mail: hk@hkeurope.com

Australia: Human Kinetics
57A Price Avenue
Lower Mitcham, South Australia 5062
08 8277 1555
e-mail: liaw@hkaustralia.com

New Zealand: Human Kinetics
Division of Sports Distributors NZ Ltd.
P.O. Box 300 226 Albany
North Shore City
Auckland
0064 9 448 1207
e-mail: info@humankinetics.co.nz

ACTION PLAN FOR

HIGH CHOLESTEROL

CONTENTS

PREFACE

Lowering your cholesterol can be a daunting task. Conflicting stories on cholesterol and health appear in the media daily, some tied to research and some tied to experience. We've put together *Action Plan for High Cholesterol* to break through this clutter, with a plan based on the latest research and breakthroughs in day-to-day treatment of cardiovascular disease.

Our focus is on giving you a better understanding of blood cholesterol, the different ways to change your blood cholesterol, and the importance of exercise in developing a healthier blood cholesterol and lipid profile. Blood cholesterol is one of the leading factors for determining your risk for cardiovascular disease or heart disease. We know absolutely that reducing blood cholesterol will lower your likelihood of developing heart disease, so this book includes different ways to lower cholesterol and develop a healthy lifestyle that will not only change your blood cholesterol profile but will increase your overall health. We will also show you how drug treatment, dietary changes, and exercise are all related in the fight to lower your heart disease risk.

What makes this book different from others? While there are many books on cholesterol and diet, this book is centered on the role of exercise in changing your cholesterol profile. You already know exercise is essential, so we're going to tell you how much is needed and how to integrate it into your daily life as part of your overall action plan. The plan is based on over 25 years of scientific research into the role of exercise on cholesterol metabolism and personal experiences from working in cardiovascular disease rehabilitation.

We've organized the book to give you everything you need to know about cholesterol as a lipid in the first chapter. Each chapter builds from there, relating cholesterol to cardiovascular disease and then discussing several ways to alter blood cholesterol, such as exercise, diet, and medications.

When you are finished reading this book, you will know that cholesterol is not all bad—it has some good qualities and is involved in various normal and healthy functions of the body. Elevated blood cholesterol is associated with abnormal bodily functions, and these characteristics in most cases lead to various diseases, mostly cardiovascular in nature.

Before reading this book, you may have heard about good and bad blood cholesterol. After reading this book, you will understand that cholesterol is carried in different forms in the blood. The good cholesterol is known in the medical community as high-density lipoprotein cholesterol (HDL-C), and the bad cholesterol is known as low-density lipoprotein cholesterol (LDL-C). You will find that some methods (medications, diet, exercise, or any combination) will modify the way your cholesterol is carried in the blood or will reduce your cholesterol. You will also learn that exercise has many positive health benefits, including an increase in good cholesterol (HDL-C) and a decrease in bad cholesterol (LDL-C). You will understand that exercise can work together with prescribed medications and a healthy diet. Most important is the chapter on exercise intervention that specifies the necessary amount of exercise for changes in blood cholesterol.

At this point you should be ready to get started in developing a better understanding of your blood cholesterol and what you can do to alter it. As you read and learn, remember that the goal of this book is to give you better knowledge of the function of blood cholesterol, the importance of cholesterol in healthy functions, and the normal blood range. Another goal for you is to learn about the different disorders of elevated cholesterol known as dyslipidemias and their link to cardiovascular disease. You will also gain information about methods other than exercise that are available to help you lower your elevated blood cholesterol. The overall intent of this book is to get you started on an exercise program to manage your blood cholesterol levels. This sounds simple, but in reality this is a challenge that will require some work. You need to remember that your definitive aim is to lower your elevated cholesterol and reduce your risk for developing premature cardiovascular disease. This goal coupled with a strong determination will better prepare you to overcome these challenges.

ACKNOWLEDGMENTS

The contributions of my students and my family made this book possible. I recognize the assistance that I received from students working with me, including Andrea Summers, Rhett Kinard, and Adam Sleister. Most importantly, I wish to extend much appreciation to my family for their support. Linda, my steadfast wife and best friend who has stood with me for more than 30 years, you are the best. Jason and Mike, your fun loving spirits have given me the encouragement to strive to be the best that I can be.

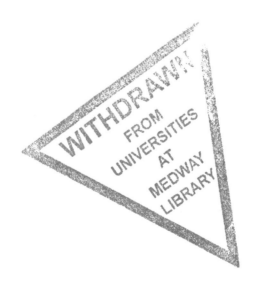

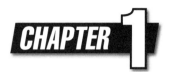

CHAPTER 1

UNDERSTANDING BLOOD CHOLESTEROL

You've picked up this book because you want to know more about blood cholesterol. Perhaps your physician has indicated that you have high blood cholesterol, or maybe your spouse or another family member has high blood cholesterol and you want to understand what that means and how to overcome this problem. Cholesterol is necessary for many of the body's functions. But when you have too much cholesterol in your body, your risk for developing certain diseases, especially heart disease, increases. This chapter provides details about cholesterol and other lipids found in the blood and the body. In addition, you will learn that you can modify blood cholesterol levels by eating a healthy diet and exercising daily. Understanding these two key concepts is essential for controlling blood cholesterol and maintaining a healthy lifestyle. On the other hand, as we will discuss in later chapters, if your blood cholesterol is still elevated even after you develop a healthy lifestyle, you may pursue other avenues such as medications or complementary or alternative therapies to help control your blood cholesterol levels.

Blood Cholesterol and Other Lipids

High cholesterol is a risk factor for heart disease, and in chapter 2 we discuss in detail the link between the two. In the meantime, remember that cholesterol is only one of several *lipids,* or *fats,* found in the blood. Though elevated cholesterol is associated with heart disease, it is modifiable, and by lowering blood cholesterol levels you can significantly reduce your risk of heart disease. In the following section, we discuss the details of cholesterol and other blood lipids, cholesterol components and their functions, and important numbers you need to know.

Cholesterol is a soft, oily substance referred to as a fat or lipid. In moderate amounts cholesterol is essential for good health, and it is incorporated in all cell walls and membranes. Cholesterol is essential in the body's process of making steroid and sex hormones such as testosterone and estrogen, and it is necessary for vitamin D synthesis. Cholesterol comes from two sources: the liver, which produces approximately 1,000 milligrams (mg) a day, and the food you eat, such as meat, egg yolks, and dairy products. As discussed in chapter 6, fruits, vegetables, grains, nuts, seeds, and other plant-based foods do not contain cholesterol, and adding these foods to a diet can reduce blood cholesterol.

If cholesterol is needed for healthy bodily function, how is cholesterol bad for you? The answer to this question is simple. A certain amount of cholesterol is important for the body. However, when blood cholesterol levels exceed 200 mg/dL (milligrams per deciliter), you become at risk for developing heart disease. In 1985 the first National Cholesterol Education Program (NCEP) recommendations were published. The basic recommendation that blood cholesterol not exceed 200 mg/dL is still in place today following an update in 2002 (NCEP 2002).

Elevated total blood cholesterol is clearly a modifiable heart disease risk factor. Many times heart attacks, bypass surgeries, angioplasties, and sudden cardiac deaths occur in people with a total cholesterol level below 200 mg/dL. A better way to estimate risk of heart disease is to know the ratio of total cholesterol to *good cholesterol*. The blood carries total cholesterol in several different forms, referred to as *lipoproteins*. These different lipoproteins are also related to risk of heart disease (we'll discuss lipoproteins in greater detail later in this chapter).

The Good, the Bad, and the Ugly

The terms *good cholesterol* (high-density lipoprotein cholesterol, or HDL-C) and *bad cholesterol* (low-density lipoprotein cholesterol, or LDL-C) are often used when discussing lipids and lipoproteins. HDL-C is called the good cholesterol because it is associated with reduced risk for premature heart disease. On the other hand, because of its association with greater risk for heart disease, LDL-C is often referred to as the bad cholesterol. Occasionally, triglycerides are referred to as the ugly lipids. This moniker is based on observations of plaque buildup on the inside lining of arterial walls, which is connected with triglyceride levels. Simply put, this buildup is not pleasant to the eye!

Other major blood lipids are triglycerides and free fatty acids (FFAs). Triglycerides serve several functions but are primarily used as a rich energy storage source. They combine three FFAs into a single molecule that is stored principally in adipose or fat tissue but is also found in all body tissues, including blood and muscle. In addition to storing fat, triglycerides are used in the construction of cell membranes. *Phospholipids* are lipids that resemble triglycerides, but instead of three FFAs grouped together, one FFA is replaced with a phosphate.

Blood Lipoproteins

Lipids do not mix well with water, just as a drop of cooking oil placed in water does not mix into the water even after stirred. Because lipids do not mix with water and therefore cannot be moved throughout the body, some other way must exist for lipids to move from place to place in the body. This movement is accomplished by joining lipids with proteins referred to as apolipoproteins (apo). There are as many as 17 different apolipoproteins, with names such as apo AI, apo AII, apo B_{48}, apo B_{100}, and apo(a). Because the new particles are the combination of lipids and proteins, they are referred to as lipoproteins. They mix with blood and other bodily fluids and thus move easily throughout the body. Lipoprotein particles contain cholesterol, triglycerides, phospholipids, and various proteins. The four general lipoprotein classifications are chylomicron, very low-density lipoprotein (VLDL), low-density lipoprotein (LDL), and high-density lipoprotein (HDL). All lipoproteins have some association with risk of heart disease (see table 1.1).

Table 1.1   Lipoproteins and Risk of Heart Disease

Lipid or lipoprotein	Relationship to heart disease
Chylomicron	Associated with increased risk
VLDL	Somewhat related to increased risk
IDL	Somewhat related to increased risk
LDL	Strongly related to increased risk
Lp(a)	Strongly related to increased risk
HDL	Strongly related to reduced risk
Cholesterol	Strongly related to increased risk
Triglyceride	Associated with increased risk

Adapted, by permission, from J.L. Durstine and P.D. Thompson, 2001, "Exercise in the treatment of lipid disorders," *Cardiology Clinics: Exercise in Secondary Prevention and Cardiac Rehabilitation* 19(3): 471-488.

• Chylomicrons are formed during digestion and absorption from the intestine, are the primary carrier of triglycerides, and are released into the blood during the hours after a meal. This time period is often referred to as the *postprandial period* (the time period immediately after and up to several hours after a meal). When you have fasted, or not eaten food, for at least 10 hours, blood chylomicron levels are nonexistent unless you have familiar hyperchylomicronemia, a rare disease. Elevated fasted chylomicron levels are associated with some increased risk of heart disease.

• VLDL particles are made mostly in the liver and are the primary transporters of postabsorptive triglyceride to all tissues in the body (the *postabsorptive period* is the time period when all blood fat originating from digestion is removed, usually 8 hours after a meal). The overproduction of triglycerides by the liver is called *hypertriglyceridemia*. Elevated fasted VLDL levels are associated with some increased risk of heart disease.

• LDL particles are made by the action of VLDL particles, a process termed the *low-density lipoprotein (LDL) receptor pathway*. As VLDL particles are broken down into lesser fragments by a blood enzyme called *lipoprotein lipase,* small amounts of triglycerides move into the tissues (e.g., fat cells, muscle cells). One portion created in this process is the LDL particle, which is the primary transporter of cholesterol to all tissues in the body. LDL-cholesterol (LDL-C) is a strong predictor of risk for heart disease.

• Lp(a) is a unique subclass of LDL because it contains apolipoprotein(a). This particle is similar in chemical composition to plasminogen, another blood protein. Plasminogen is involved in a series of chemical reactions that break up blood clots. Because Lp(a) is chemically similar to plasminogen, it prevents plasminogen from breaking up blood clots. As a result, the blood-clotting process is enhanced, thus facilitating the final stages leading to a heart attack. Generally, blood Lp(a) levels greater than 20 to 25 mg/dL are associated with a greatly increased risk for premature heart disease. Lp(a), unfortunately, is an inherited trait and is treatable only by medication.

• HDL particles are made in the liver and small intestine and are released into the blood. HDL functions in a different movement process, termed *reverse cholesterol transport,* from that of the other lipoproteins. In this process, HDL collects cholesterol from the peripheral tissues and moves it to the liver, where it is removed from the blood and eliminated from the body. Because HDL moves cholesterol back to the liver where it can be carried out of the body, it has become known as good cholesterol and is negatively associated with risk for developing heart disease. Thus, having high levels of HDL-C is a goal that all individuals should strive to achieve.

Lipoprotein Transport Pathways

Together, blood lipids, lipoproteins, and the cardiovascular system provide for the complex movement and exchange of cholesterol and triglycerides among the intestine, liver, and all body tissues. Though several lipoprotein pathways exist, we'll discuss two distinct pathways here (LDL receptor pathway and reverse cholesterol transport) that, when genetically or environmentally disturbed, result in altered blood lipid and lipoprotein profiles and modified risk of heart disease.

LDL Receptor Pathway

The LDL receptor pathway consists of a series of steps to deliver cholesterol and triglycerides to all the body tissues. Dietary fat, also called *exogenous fat,* is digested by the small intestine and absorbed as cholesterol, triglycerides, and fatty acids. These lipids combine with proteins and become chylomicrons, which are released into the blood. Once in the blood, chylomicrons move throughout the body, but they are continually being broken down. As part of the chylomicron breakdown, triglycerides and FFAs are released where they can move into body cells. Eventually, blood chylomicrons become much smaller and are transformed into VLDL particles. The liver is another source of VLDL, which is the primary transporter of *endogenous fat,* or fat made by the liver. Whether the VLDL originated from dietary fat or fat made in the liver, VLDL breakdown continues until the much smaller LDL particles are formed. In the transformation from VLDL to LDL, triglycerides are removed and cholesterol added until the smaller LDL (the primary transporter of blood cholesterol) is formed. All body cells have surface receptors that move LDL-C inside the cell where it is used for many cellular functions such as membrane development and steroid hormone synthesis. Under normal circumstances, when cell cholesterol reaches a certain level, further cholesterol uptake and synthesis are halted.

Genetic and environmental factors can interrupt the normal function of the LDL receptor pathway, and when this pathway functions improperly, excess blood cholesterol is thought to accumulate on the lining of arterial walls. After some time, perhaps years, of lipid accumulation, the passageway of the artery narrows. When coronary arteries narrow, blood delivery to the heart is reduced. Delivery of nutriments like oxygen is also reduced or even stopped. This condition is commonly referred to as heart disease or *coronary artery disease* and can lead to a heart attack.

The C in HDL-C and LDL-C

Lipoprotein abbreviations such as HDL and LDL often include the letter *C* (for example, HDL-C), which stands for cholesterol. It simply means that cholesterol is associated with that lipoprotein. Sometimes *TG* is used, which refers to the triglyceride associated with that lipoprotein (for example, VLDL-TG).

Reverse Cholesterol Transport

Reverse cholesterol transport involves a series of chemical reactions necessary to collect excess cholesterol from peripheral tissues and move it back to the liver, where it is removed from the body. This transport can occur through several different biological pathways. Most scientists believe that blood HDL particles interact with other lipoproteins such as VLDL and LDL to collect excessive cholesterol and triglycerides. During this reverse transport process HDL grows until it is much larger, or mature, and can no longer collect any more lipids. The mature HDL moves to the liver, where the cholesterol and triglycerides are removed. The HDL particles minus cholesterol and triglycerides are now ready to return to the blood and circulate, collecting more cholesterol. As with the LDL receptor pathway, genetic and environmental factors affect the reverse transport process. For example, regular exercise usually results in an increased blood HDL-C, which in turn reduces the risk of premature heart disease.

Lipid Ratios

Lipid ratios such as the ratio of total cholesterol to HDL-C (total cholesterol/HDL-C) and LDL-C to HDL-C (LDL-C/HDL-C) are strong predictors of heart disease risk, though the total cholesterol/HDL-C ratio is the better predictor. In any case, both ratios use a blood lipid measure that is directly related to increased risk of heart disease (total cholesterol or LDL-C) and contrasts it with a blood lipid value that is associated with decreased risk of heart disease (HDL-C). Consider the following example. If your blood total cholesterol is 230 and HDL-C is 30, your ratio of heart disease risk is 230/30. By dividing 230 by 30, we obtain a value for the lipid risk ratio, which is 7.67. This number is higher than the NCEP-recommended value of 4.5 for men and 4.0 for women. In this case, steps should be taken to lower the total cholesterol and raise HDL-C levels. On the other hand, a total cholesterol value of 175 and an HDL-C value of 48 would yield a value of 3.65. This risk ratio is very healthy for both men and women and is associated with lower risk of heart disease.

Genetic Factors Influencing Blood Cholesterol

Through proper exercise and nutritional counseling and adherence to a healthy lifestyle, most people can control their blood cholesterol, but due to genetic conditions some individuals require medications to lower their blood cholesterol. Even responses to dietary changes are influenced by genetic factors. For example, some people have low blood cholesterol despite consuming a diet high in saturated fat, being obese, and getting little exercise. At the same time, some people have an unacceptable blood cholesterol and lipoprotein profile despite careful attention to health-related factors. Likewise, the effects of exercise on blood cholesterol and lipoproteins can be influenced by genetics. For example, various apolipoprotein E (apo E) genotypic variations are known to exist, and people with the apo E2 genotype who also participate regularly in exercise have a greater beneficial change in their lipid and lipoprotein profile than people with another apo E genotype. This evidence supports the idea that the effect of exercise on the blood lipid and lipoprotein profile is, at least in part, genetically regulated.

Although much is known about the association of genetic disorders and abnormal lipid and lipoprotein levels, only two relatively common genetic disorders associated with premature heart disease are addressed

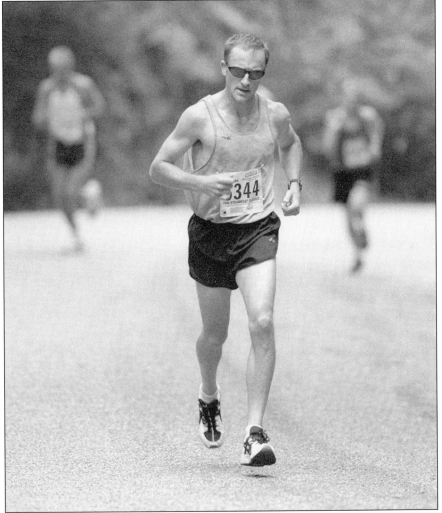

© Human Kinetics

Lifestyle changes such as exercise and a healthy diet help to lower cholesterol, though genetics also contribute to the equation.

here: *familial heterozygous hypercholesterolemia* and *familial dysbetalipo-proteinemia,* or type III hyperlipidemia.

Familial heterozygous hypercholesterolemia is a condition resulting in the inability of the LDL receptor pathway to deliver cholesterol to cells. This condition has many potential areas where problems could occur. For instance, the LDL receptors found on all cells may not function properly, or the blood LDL-C particles may not have the proper apolipoproteins to bind to the cell's LDL receptor. Whatever the reason, a person with this condition has elevated blood LDL-C and is at high risk for premature heart disease. In addition, risk of premature heart disease is related to the degree of defects in the LDL-C pathway and environmental influences such as poor dietary habits. An unhealthy lifestyle coupled with genetic factors can work synergistically to worsen heart disease risk.

Type III hyperlipidemia is highly associated with premature heart disease and is characterized by cholesterol-enriched VLDL and LDL particles. Again, different potential genetic defects are involved, including overproduction of endogenous cholesterol and triglycerides and the cells' inability to move cholesterol inside. Environmental factors such as poor dietary habits, obesity, mild hypothyroidism, diabetes, and lack of regular exercise complicate this condition.

Determining Your Lipid and Lipoprotein Profile

A blood lipid and lipoprotein profile that includes triglycerides, cholesterol, cholesterol associated with HDL and LDL, and blood glucose is obtained from a simple blood test. The general belief is that anyone with a family history of heart disease or diabetes should have these tests completed early in life. When family history of heart disease is strong, even the children should have these blood tests. The tests can be completed in a physician's office and usually require a 10- to 14-hour overnight fast. Drinking water is permitted, but if you smoke, you should abstain from smoking until after the test. Fasting is not required for total cholesterol and HDL-C measurement, but it is required for triglyceride and blood glucose measurements. Fasting for 10 or more hours eliminates any blood glucose or triglycerides formed as a result of dietary intake and digestive absorption.

Levels of blood lipids and lipoproteins are affected by a variety of circumstances. Alcohol and sugar increase triglyceride levels, while a high-fat diet, the common cold, emotional stress, and the menstrual cycle can affect the results of the blood test. HDL-C and triglycerides are altered by alcohol intake and even a single exercise session.

Another consideration is the body's ability or inability to clear fat from the blood after a meal. The period of time after a meal where lipid levels are elevated over premeal values is referred to as postprandial *lipemia*. Exaggerated or prolonged postprandial lipemia is the increased time needed after a meal to remove blood lipids. Recent scientific information suggests that a reduced postprandial lipemia is associated with reduced risk of heart disease (Poppitt 2005). Postprandial lipemia is reduced with regular exercise.

LDL-C currently cannot be measured in the physician's office. Though it is possible to directly measure LDL-C, this analysis is a long and costly process and requires expensive equipment. Instead, LDL-C is usually calculated by determining fasting triglyceride, total cholesterol, and HDL-C values and using them in the following equation:

$$LDL\text{-}C = (\text{total cholesterol} - HDL\text{-}C) - \text{triglyceride}/5$$

Heart disease risk is very low for LDL-C values less than 100 mg/dL but increases for values from 100 to 130. After blood values of 130 mg/dL are reached, heart disease risk grows at enormous rates.

So what are the lipid and lipoprotein values that you should remember? In the past a variety of blood cholesterol values according to age and gender were used to determine your heart disease risk. Now, however, the NCEP recommends some simple values to remember. Triglycerides should be less than 150 mg/dL, total cholesterol less than 200 mg/dL, LDL-C less than 100 mg/dL, and HDL-C greater than 40 mg/dL for men and 45 for women. See table 1.2 for a summary of these values.

Table 1.2 NCEP Recommendations

Lipid or lipoprotein	Recommended value
Triglyceride	Less than 150 mg/dL
Cholesterol	Less than 200 mg/dL
LDL-C	Less than 100 mg/dL
HDL-C	Greater than 40 mg/dL for men and 45 mg/dL for women

From the National Heart, Lung and Blood Institute and the National Institutes of Health (NIH), a section of the US Department of Health and Human Services. http://www.nhlbi.nih.gov/chd/

Information gained from a blood lipid and lipoprotein profile is beneficial in establishing risk of heart disease and also in starting a therapeutic lifestyle-change program to reduce the likelihood of developing heart disease. To better understand actual lipid and lipoprotein profile values, consider the following two examples. The first example is a blood test with the following information: triglycerides = 260, total cholesterol = 240, HDL-C = 35, and blood glucose = 200. Using the equation previously discussed, we can calculate LDL-C.

$$LDL\text{-}C = (240 - 35) - 260/5$$
$$LDL\text{-}C = 205 - 52$$
$$LDL\text{-}C = 153$$

Any person with these lipid and lipoprotein profile values would be at great risk for developing premature heart disease. The triglyceride levels are not quite double the 150 mg/dL recommended by NCEP. Total cholesterol is well over the recommended level of 200 mg/dL, LDL-C is well over the recommended level of 100 mg/dL, HDL-C is less than the recommended value of 40 mg/dL, and the TC/HDL-C ratio is 6.86, well over the recommended value of 4.5. Blood glucose is also well over the recommended value of 110 mg/dL, and this person is suspected of having diabetes as well as being at risk for premature heart disease.

Let's consider a second example. In this case, the blood lipid and lipoprotein profile contains the following information: triglycerides = 150, total cholesterol = 180, HDL-C = 45, and blood glucose = 90. The TC/HDL-C ratio is 4.0. The calculation for LDL-C is as follows:

$$LDL\text{-}C = (180 - 45) - 150/5$$
$$LDL\text{-}C = 135 - 30$$
$$LDL\text{-}C = 105$$

Heart disease risk for the person in this example is much different from that for the person in the first example. All lipid, lipoprotein, and ratio values are well within acceptable ranges. Blood glucose is also in an acceptable range. This individual's overall risk of developing heart disease is low.

Reducing Cholesterol and Ensuring a Healthier Heart

As you'll see in chapter 2, many factors associated with high cholesterol and heart disease overlap. The best way to improve your cholesterol and lipoprotein profile is to focus on reducing factors that negatively affect cholesterol, concentrating especially on the factors that are the easiest to change: lifestyle factors such as being overweight and being sedentary. Current recommendations for managing blood lipid and lipoprotein values have been provided by the NCEP (see table 1.2 on page 9). Dietary modifications, weight loss, and exercise are recommended as initial therapeutic lifestyle changes. Other environmental factors such as smoking and stress management also affect lipid and lipoprotein concentrations. When each of these factors is positively altered through therapeutic lifestyle changes such as eating food low in saturated fat, starting an exercise program, quitting smoking, or reducing daily stress, the blood lipid and lipoprotein profile is altered in a positive direction. More important, these positive lifestyle changes can work synergistically with each other, bringing about even greater blood lipid and lipoprotein changes. This book focuses on exercise and healthy eating as paths to weight loss and lower blood cholesterol levels.

Dietary modification and weight loss.   Positive changes in blood cholesterol, triglycerides, and lipoproteins result from reductions in cholesterol consumption and percentage of dietary fat as well as changes in the type of fat consumed (see chapter 6). Not only does the reduction of dietary fat reduce the amount of fat absorbed by the digestive system, but low dietary fat can reduce the amount of fat that the liver produces, which can further reduce blood cholesterol. Keep in mind that diets that are low in fat and high in carbohydrate can also lower blood HDL-C while increasing triglyceride levels. Remember also that weight loss achieved by caloric restriction is associated with lower blood cholesterol and LDL-C. Consequently, reductions in dietary fat and weight loss achieved by caloric restriction magnify the beneficial blood lipid and lipoprotein changes that result from exercise. Many overweight individuals who have elevated blood cholesterol, triglyceride, and LDL-C levels and reduced HDL-C levels will benefit from therapeutic lifestyle changes. Overweight persons who restrict dietary fat, reduce caloric intake, and participate in regular exercise can positively affect their blood lipid and lipoprotein profiles.

Exercise.   As discussed in chapter 3, regular exercise will reduce blood triglyceride and LDL-C while increasing HDL-C levels. When an exercise program, a weight-loss program, and a low-fat diet are started at the same time, they work synergistically to result in greater positive lipid and lipoprotein profile changes, including reductions in blood cholesterol.

Summary

Cholesterol is a critical heart disease risk factor that is influenced by both genetic and environmental conditions. If your blood cholesterol is elevated, there *is* something you can do to reduce your cholesterol and the way your cholesterol is transported by lipoproteins in the blood. The remainder of this book considers the role of cholesterol in the development of heart disease and how lifestyle changes can positively modify blood cholesterol and lipoproteins.

UNDERSTANDING BLOOD CHOLESTEROL

☐ Learn the functions and recommended levels of

- cholesterol,
- triglycerides,
- free fatty acids,
- chylomicrons,
- VLDL,
- LDL, and
- HDL.

☐ Learn about the problems that lipids and lipoproteins cause when their levels are not optimal.

☐ Understand how cholesterol is moved throughout the body, and how the ratios of total cholesterol to HDL-C and LDL-C to HDL-C act as predictors of heart disease risk.

☐ Be aware that genetic factors play a role in blood cholesterol levels.

☐ Become familiar with the terminology involved in the lipid and lipoprotein profile, how these numbers are generated, and details to keep in mind before having your cholesterol levels tested.

☐ Be encouraged that unhealthy cholesterol levels can be improved through lifestyle modifications such as exercise and healthy eating. Read on to find out more!

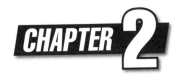

CHAPTER 2

LINKING CHOLESTEROL AND HEART DISEASE

oronary artery disease (CAD) or coronary heart disease (CHD) are terms often used to refer to heart disease—a disease that for many decades has been the number one cause of death for men and women in the United States. Heart attacks account for 46 percent of all deaths in Western countries. In the United States, each year approximately 1.5 million people have heart attacks, and 500,000 deaths occur (AHA 2005). Each year doctors perform more than 600,000 coronary artery bypass surgeries and more than 500,000 coronary angioplasties. Heart disease isn't just a man's disease; heart attacks, strokes, and other cardiovascular diseases are devastating to women as well. Many women believe that cancer is a greater threat, but that assumption is wrong. Nearly twice as many women in the United States die from heart disease and stroke than from all forms of cancer combined, including breast cancer (AHA 2005); see also the sidebar on page 14.

Researchers and doctors maintain that heart disease is associated with many different genetic and lifestyle risk factors. Over time, the list of genetic and environmental risk factors contributing to the development of heart disease has gotten longer. For almost everyone the factors that lead to heart disease appear threatening. Fortunately, once many of these risk factors are detected, steps can be taken to reduce their presence, and when that happens, the risk for the disease is also lowered and the disease process itself is slowed or perhaps even stopped. In other words, heart disease in most cases is preventable. This chapter explains normal artery function, the development of heart disease, and the risk factors for heart disease, including high cholesterol.

Men, Women, and Heart Disease

Men have a much higher rate of heart disease than premenopausal women do; onset of heart disease lags behind nearly 10 to 20 years for women. However, heart disease remains the leading cause of overall death for both men and women. The delay of onset in women is thought to be related in part to estrogen, a female hormone. After menopause, when estrogen levels fall, heart disease rates for women close in on those for men. The role of hormone replacement therapy (HRT) in decreasing the risk of heart disease in postmenopausal women is still unclear. Clinical research trials have found HRT to be effective in raising HDL-C values and lowering LDL-C, total blood cholesterol, and fibrinogen levels, but the benefits of HRT, as far as reducing the risk of heart disease, have recently been viewed in light of the increased likelihood of some forms of cancer.

Coronary Vascular System

The heart is like any other organ in that it needs a continuous flow of blood in order to function. As a result, the heart has its own blood supply, the coronary vascular system, which is made up of arteries, capillaries, and veins. Blood flows through two primary *coronary arteries* (the right and left coronary arteries) into the three layers of the heart: the endocardium, the myocardium, and the epicardium. The two coronary arteries branch from the *aorta,* which is the largest artery in the body (see figure 2.1). The right coronary artery supplies blood to the right side of the heart while the left coronary artery supplies blood to the left side of the heart. The coronary arteries divide into smaller arteries, and each time the arteries divide they reach deeper into the layers of the heart. Eventually, the arteries divide into the smallest arteries, called arterioles, which lead to the capillaries. The capillaries provide a connection to the veins, and they are the point where nutriments such as oxygen are exchanged for waste products such as carbon dioxide. Inside the capillaries in the area closest to the arterioles is the point where oxygen moves into the tissue, and at the farthest end of the capillaries in the area close to the veins is the point where carbon dioxide produced in the tissues moves into the capillaries. The veins then return the blood to the heart. The coronary vascular system is a complex blood supply system, and if reduction of blood delivery to any part of the heart occurs, oxygen delivery is also reduced. Without oxygen, heart tissue will die.

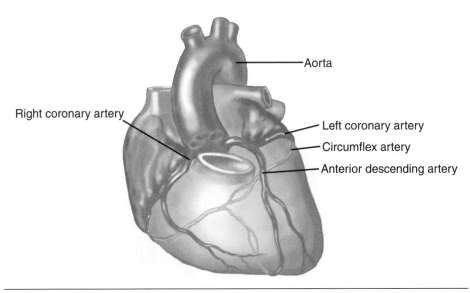

Figure 2.1 Coronary vascular system.

Normal Function of Arteries

The coronary arteries, like all arteries, have an opening through which blood flows. This open area is known as the *lumen.* Arteries also have three distinct layers. The innermost layer is called the *intima,* the outermost layer is the *adventitia,* and the layer in between the two is the *media* (see figure 2.2). The intimal layer, which is the layer next to where blood flows, is lined with a single layer of cells called the *endothelium* that acts as a barrier between the blood and the other artery layers. Cells found in the arterial walls contain many receptors, including ones for LDL molecules and other growth factors.

Arterial wall cells also produce substances that are capable of a wide variety of actions, such as dissolving blood clots. One such substance produced by the endothelium is *nitric oxide.* This substance causes the artery to widen its lumen and allow for greater blood flow. Nitric oxide has several other important functions including inhibiting platelet formation, platelet attachment to the arterial wall, and suppressing formation of blood clots. Nitric oxide also controls smooth muscle cell (SMC) proliferation (increase in number) within the arterial wall and SMC movement from one arterial wall layer to another. All of these actions are necessary in maintaining normal endothelium development and function.

The LDL receptor pathway is the process for moving cholesterol into cells. LDL receptors are found on the surface of all human cells.

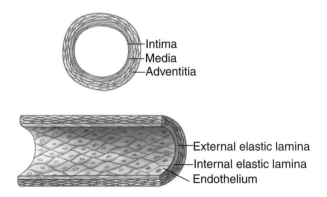

Figure 2.2 Normal coronary arterial wall.

These receptors bind with LDL particles found in the blood or other body fluids. Once LDL particles containing cholesterol join with the cell's LDL receptor, they are taken into the cell where the cholesterol is either released for cellular use or stored. Michael S. Brown and Joseph L. Goldstein of the University of Texas Health Science Center at Dallas won the 1985 Nobel Prize in physiology and medicine for discovering this key metabolic pathway for cholesterol. This discovery revolutionized scientific knowledge about regulating metabolism of cholesterol and treating diseases caused by abnormally elevated blood cholesterol levels. One of Brown and Goldstein's many important discoveries is that the human body's normal cholesterol production stops when the cholesterol within a cell reaches a certain level. When this process is not working normally, excessive amounts of blood cholesterol develop. It is this excessive blood cholesterol and the reduced cholesterol removal that are the most common factors contributing to *atherosclerosis*. Current knowledge points to blood cholesterol, particularly the LDL-C form, as the lipid that accumulates most in the atherosclerotic lesion. Excessive blood cholesterol accumulates when LDL-C endothelial levels are high or cell cholesterol breakdown and removal are impaired.

Heart Disease

Arteriosclerosis refers to a group of cardiovascular disorders that cause arterial walls to thicken and harden. Atherosclerosis is a form of arteriosclerosis and is associated with plaque formation on the inner lining of arteries. Plaque is composed of fats, mostly cholesterol, but also triglycerides and phospholipids as well as other substances including platelets, fibrin, calcium, and connective tissue. Plaque growth, which occurs gradually over a long period of time, injures the lining of the arterial wall (endothelium). Eventually, the affected endothelial tissue undergoes *necrosis,* or dies, and an overgrowth of connective tissue develops around the injured area, forming a scar. This scarring promotes further buildup of plaque. After years of plaque accumulation, the passage for blood flow becomes quite narrow, and a blood clot *(thrombus)* forms on the surface of the plaque, blocking and even stopping blood flow through the artery. Plaque buildup and clot formation can occur in any of the arteries found in the body, but when it happens in the coronary arteries, the disease process is referred to as coronary artery disease (CAD) or heart disease. As plaque builds up and stops blood flow through the coronary arteries, delivery of oxygen to the heart stops and a heart attack, or *myocardial infarction,* occurs. The larger the area affected by the lack of blood, the larger the heart attack and the greater the necrosis.

Atherosclerosis

Several hypotheses exist that explain the process of atherosclerosis. The two hypotheses with the most scientific support suggest that atherosclerosis is caused either by injury response or by inflammation.

Normal endothelial function promotes arterial blood flow to meet the surrounding tissue's need for oxygen. At the same time it protects the artery against atherosclerosis by regulating blood clot formation and smooth muscle cell (SMC) proliferation. However, when the endothelial lining of the arterial wall is injured, normal endothelial function is interrupted and the injured lining is repaired. The repair process leads to the release of substances such as platelet-derived growth factor, which augments arterial wall production of connective tissue and SMC proliferation. According to the *injury response hypothesis,* this repair process also initiates plaque buildup and atherosclerosis.

The *inflammation hypothesis* suggests that inflammation occurs in the endothelium. This inflammation may be the result of many factors, and it initiates the immune inflammatory response. One of the first responses is for *monocytes,* a type of white blood cell, to attach to the endothelial layer of the arterial wall and eventually move into the intimal layer. When the monocytes attach to the arterial wall, they begin to gather excessive cholesterol. As the monocytes accumulate cholesterol, they convert into *macrophages;* this conversion is the start of atherosclerosis. Macrophages increase LDL-C oxidation, which can enhance their entry into intima cells. A macrophage also has scavenger receptors that are capable of binding with LDL-C and moving these particles inside the cell. All of these actions lead to excessive cholesterol accumulation inside the artery.

Plaque buildup is most likely a result of both injury and inflammation. Regardless, both hypotheses suggest that the attachment of monocytes to the endothelium promotes production and release of platelet-derived growth factor. With the deposit of platelets, the endothelium begins to accumulate cholesterol. Monocytes attach to the endothelial layer and then are incorporated into the intimal layer. This sequence of events promotes SMC and fibroblast movement into the intimal layer as well. All of these events cause the collection of excessive cholesterol as well as other lipids into early atherosclerotic lesions referred to as fatty streaks. Fatty streaks continue to grow by attracting more connective tissue, SMC, cholesterol, and other lipids. As the fatty streaks grow over time, they become known as raised plaque, or *fibrolipid plaque.* Raised plaque is linked to increases in fibrous tissue and the development of a fibrous cap over the cholesterol-filled core, and it is responsible for the narrowing of the lumen opening and thus impairment of blood flow. During the final stage of atherosclerosis, a blood clot forms around the plaque. Blood clots develop either from bleeding in the area of the plaque buildup or from plaques that rupture.

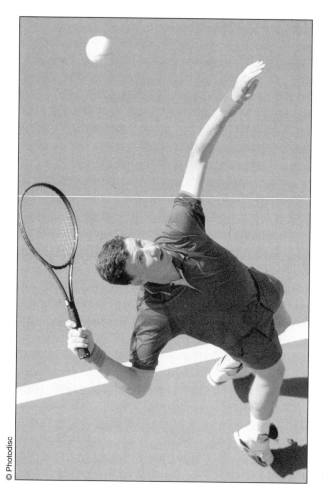

© Photodisc

Adding exercise and physical activity to your life is the best way to avoid one of the risk factors for heart disease—a sedentary lifestyle.

Plaque Rupture

Plaque may be soft or hard. In either case, as the plaque builds up in the coronary arteries, blood flow to the heart tissue is reduced, which means the heart receives less oxygen and chest pain and a heart attack are more likely to result. *Soft plaque* is susceptible to rupture and can lead to blood clot formation and ultimately a heart attack. It can take years for soft plaque to turn into *hard plaque* with a fibrous cap. However, new scientific findings suggest that many heart attacks are actually caused by soft plaque because it is vulnerable to rupture. Cholesterol, especially elevated LDL-C levels, contributes to instability and rupturing of plaque. In contrast, HDL-C plays a role in restricting SMC growth and adding to plaque stability. Thus, scientists believe that lowering blood LDL-C levels and increasing HDL-C levels is helpful in stabilizing soft plaque and reducing rupture.

The strength and integrity of the fibrous cap overlying the LDL-C–rich core determine lesion stability. Plaque prone to rupture has a thin fibrous cap, whereas stable plaque has a thicker fibrous cap. Forces contributing to plaque rupture include elevated LDL-C, increased blood pressure, and nicotine from smoking. Immune system responses also play an important role in plaque rupture. For example, macrophages release enzymes and other elements that erode the plaque. Upon plaque rupture, circulating platelets quickly come in contact with the plaque, providing the groundwork for a blood clot to develop.

Finally, soft plaques blocking less than 50 percent of an artery were in the past not viewed as a serious concern. These types of plaques were thought to take years to grow in size and completely block the blood flow through the vessel. However, present scientific information suggests that many of these soft plaques are more likely to rupture, causing a blood clot to form that will block blood flow and result in a heart attack. Therefore, not all advanced hard plaques are responsible for heart attacks; as previously mentioned, heart attacks can be the result of formation and rupture of soft plaque. This explains why some people suffering a heart attack for the first time do not have a history of heart disease or other signs and symptoms such as chest pain.

Risk Factors for Heart Disease

The process by which heart disease develops has long been thought to begin during childhood and advance at a slow rate throughout adulthood. However, recent research suggests that the disease can also start later in life and progress at faster rates. Whether advancing slowly or quickly or starting early or late in life, heart disease reduces the inside size of the artery as well as the functioning of the lining of the coronary arteries. As a result, the delivery of valuable nutriments such as oxygen is dramatically reduced, and in the worst-case scenario, if blood flow stops, oxygen delivery to the heart tissue stops, leading to a heart attack.

The risk of heart disease can be reduced, but prevention of heart disease is most successful when started early. Identification and reduction of risk factors should be started early in life. This process of preventing a heart attack is referred to as primary prevention. At the same time, when persons have already suffered a heart attack, steps can be taken to reduce the risk for another. Coronary artery bypass surgery, balloon angioplasty, and lifestyle interventions in this case are referred to as secondary prevention.

Regarding slowing the onset or occurrence of heart disease, questions that come to mind include who should be concerned about prevention of heart disease, what the risk factors are, whether there is more than one risk factor, and when prevention of heart disease should start. These questions are important, and everyone should be concerned about knowing the answers. As already stated, heart disease is the leading cause of premature death in the United States. Unfortunately, most people are unaware of this fact. Even more unfortunate is the fact that many people believe heart disease won't happen to them. But because this disease is the leading cause of death in the United States, many people are in one way or another affected by it.

In the last 50 years a number of specific risk factors for heart disease have been identified, and you should be able to identify your own personal factors that increase your risk of developing premature heart disease. Once you know your risk factors, you should take certain steps to reduce them. Following is a list of common risk factors, including high cholesterol, which we will discuss in greater detail later in the chapter.

Common Risk Factors for Heart Disease

- Family history of heart disease
- Being a male over the age of 45
- Being a female over the age of 55 or a female having undergone premature menopause (e.g., as a result of surgery)
- Elevated cholesterol levels
- High blood pressure (hypertension)
- Cigarette smoking
- Sedentary lifestyle
- Obesity
- Diabetes
- Stress

Emerging Risk Factors for Heart Disease

- Elevated levels of lipoprotein(a), also known as Lp(a) (pronounced as "L-P-little a")
- Homocysteine
- C-reactive protein (CRP)
- Metabolic syndrome, or insulin resistance

Framingham Heart Study

Coronary artery plaque is composed mostly of cholesterol, as well as triglycerides, phospholipids, and substances such as platelets, fibrin, calcium, and connective tissue. Of these substances, total blood cholesterol and LDL-C are associated the most with heart disease and have received intensive scientific evaluation by several prominent clinical investigations. Of these clinical studies the Framingham Heart Study is the most recognized.

In 1948, the Framingham Heart Study in conjunction with the National Heart Institute (now known as the National Heart, Lung, and Blood Institute, or NHLBI) started a long-term research project. The objective of the Framingham Heart Study was to identify the common contributing factors to cardiovascular disease by following the development of the disease over many years in a large group of participants who had not yet acquired observable heart disease signs or symptoms. Since the beginning of the 19th century American death rates from heart disease have steadily increased, but when the Framingham Heart Study began, little was known about the general causes of heart disease. Because of the Framingham Heart Study, the role of blood cholesterol in the development of heart disease is now better understood and is accepted by physicians as a major risk factor.

The study proved a tremendous success, and at the top of its long list of accomplishments was the establishment of the relationship between blood cholesterol and heart disease. Just as important, this study showed that the cholesterol associated with lipoproteins is multifaceted in its association with heart disease. For example, the project established a strong positive association between LDL-C and heart disease as well as a strong protective HDL-C effect. The Framingham Heart Study findings changed the way we look at this disease and led to the development of educational opportunities to increase awareness of heart disease. As a result many more Americans are being treated for high blood cholesterol and high blood pressure and are learning about the dangers of smoking. Most important is the study's effect on physicians—it caused them to place greater emphasis on the prevention, detection, and treatment of heart disease in the earliest stages of development.

Lipids and Lipoproteins As Risk Factors

Thanks to projects like the Framingham Heart Study and similar clinical studies, the connection between elevated blood cholesterol and the development of heart disease is well established. Treating elevated blood cholesterol, high blood pressure, and diabetes; stopping smoking; and regularly participating in physical activity are the primary means to fight heart disease. Therapeutic lifestyle-change programs and lipid-lowering medications that promote exercise, weight loss, and reduction of dietary fat are all associated with positive changes in the blood lipid and lipoprotein profile that reduce the risk of heart disease.

Cholesterol

As we've mentioned several times, elevated blood cholesterol levels are associated with a greater likelihood for developing premature heart disease (see figure 2.3), and by lowering your blood cholesterol you reduce your risk of heart disease. As discussed in chapter 1, cholesterol is manufactured by the liver and is also obtained from food. Cholesterol is necessary for normal bodily functions such as development of cell walls and synthesis of steroid hormones; the problem is having too much cholesterol. The Framingham Heart Study helped define the critical blood cholesterol level for increased risk of heart disease as greater than 200 mg/dL. Individuals with total blood cholesterol levels exceeding 300 mg/dL have three to five times the risk of heart disease than individuals with a blood cholesterol level of 200 mg/dL. However, note that only 3 to 5 percent of the Framingham Heart Study participants had a blood cholesterol level greater than 300 mg/dL. Persons with blood cholesterol over 300 mg/dL most likely have a genetic problem, and the primary way to manage a genetic problem is with medications, with supplemental exercise and diet.

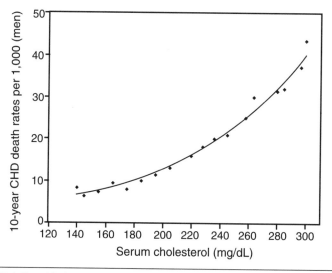

Figure 2.3 Relationship between blood cholesterol level and heart disease rate.
From the National Institutes of Health (NIH), a section of the US Department of Health and Human Services.

Triglycerides

The question of whether elevated triglyceride levels in the blood lead to heart disease is controversial. While most doctors believe that an abnormally high triglyceride level is a risk factor for heart disease, it is difficult to conclusively prove that elevated triglycerides by itself can cause atherosclerosis. However, most clinicians recognize that elevated blood triglycerides are associated with other conditions that increase the risk of heart disease, including obesity, low HDL-C levels, insulin resistance, poorly controlled diabetes, and elevated levels of small, dense LDL-C particles. The link between blood triglyceride levels and heart disease tends to weaken or even disappear with higher blood HDL-C levels. Though a strong positive association between high triglyceride values and heart disease has not been clearly defined, the NCEP sets accepted triglyceride levels at less than 150 mg/dL.

LDL-C

Present research suggests that knowing your blood cholesterol levels is important, but knowing the way blood cholesterol is spread among the various blood lipoproteins is equally important. Most of the cholesterol associated with heart disease risk is explained by LDL-C levels. As we discussed in chapter 1, LDL-C is known as the bad cholesterol, and several LDL forms exist. One form is oxidized LDL-C, a major factor in arterial plaque development. Oxidation occurs when LDL-C comes in contact with *free radicals,* which are highly unstable, reactive oxygen molecules circulating in the blood. Oxidized LDL-C readily adheres to the endothelial lining of the arteries and is much more likely to form plaque. Oxidized LDL can cause other damage as well, including damage to the lipid membranes of the arterial cells. Because oxidized LDL-C is found in significantly greater amounts in arterial plaque and because it plays a major role in the formation of artery-blocking plaque, oxidized LDL-C is a dangerous factor.

LDL-C particle size is another consideration and is represented by the LDL patterns A and B, which refer to the size of the particles. Scientists and physicians believe that small LDL-C particles pose a greater risk for developing atherosclerosis and heart attacks than the absolute blood LDL-C level. LDL-C particle size is primarily inherited. A special blood test called gradient gel electrophoresis is used to measure particle size and determine whether you have LDL-C pattern A or pattern B. Individuals with pattern A have large, buoyant LDL-C particles with normal blood HDL-C and triglyceride levels, and such people are less likely to have heart disease. On the other hand, individuals with pattern B have predominantly small, dense LDL-C particles. Pattern B is frequently associated with low HDL-C levels, elevated triglyceride levels, and the tendency to develop type 2 diabetes. Individuals with pattern B are also more likely to develop postprandial hyperlipidemia or high triglyceride levels after a fatty meal, and they have three to five times the risk of having a heart attack. LDL-C pattern B is likely the most important cause of heart disease in people with normal or near-normal total LDL-C levels. Researchers believe that the smaller LDL-C particles are more easily oxidized and as a result are found in greater amounts in plaque. Others believe that because the LDL-C particles are small they move easily into the endothelial layer, causing plaque buildup.

Regardless, higher levels of LDL-C, especially pattern B particles, combined with other risk factors such as hypertension or diabetes increase the risk of heart disease, heart attack, and stroke. Lowering your blood cholesterol and LDL-C levels reduces your risk of heart disease, even if your blood LDL-C levels are average. The NCEP recommends reducing LDL-C levels to 130 mg/dL or less in individuals without known heart disease and to 100 mg/dL or less in patients with known coronary heart disease (those who have already had a heart attack or have undergone coronary artery angioplasty or bypass surgery). More recent reports recommend LDL-C levels of less than 70 mg/dL in persons with known heart disease (Grundy et al. 2004). These types of aggressive measures for lowering cholesterol have been successful in slowing heart disease in the coronary arteries.

HDL-C

We have established that if your blood cholesterol and LDL-C levels are elevated you are more likely to have heart disease, whereas if your HDL-C is elevated you are less likely to have heart disease. Epidemiologic studies suggest that for every 1 mg/dL your HDL-C levels increase, you achieve a 2 percent decrease in heart disease risk if you are a man and a 3 percent decrease if you are a woman. Thus, the higher your HDL-C levels, the better. Because the relationship between HDL-C and risk of heart disease extends over a wide range of HDL-C levels, the NCEP has established three HDL-C categories: low is less than 40 mg/dL, normal is 40 to 60 mg/dL, and high is greater than 60 mg/dL. The NCEP classifies low HDL cholesterol as a major risk factor. Conversely, a high level is called a negative, or protective, factor. While high HDL-C offsets some of the risk that comes from having high LDL-C, low LDL-C does not eliminate the risk imparted by low HDL-C. The risk of heart attack in both men and women is highest with lower HDL-C levels and elevated blood cholesterol and LDL-C levels. However, if you have low HDL-C levels (less than 40 mg/dL), you are at high risk for heart disease, regardless of your total cholesterol level. On the other hand, if you have high total blood cholesterol, your risk of a heart attack is lower when you have higher levels of HDL-C.

Though the epidemiologic links between heart disease risk and HDL-C levels exist, we do not fully understand the underlying reasons for elevated HDL-C and lower heart disease risk. Some researchers believe that high HDL-C levels weaken the role of LDL-C in developing heart disease. If this is true, low HDL-C levels may actually encourage heart disease. The HDL-C link to heart disease risk may simply be that a low HDL-C level often indicates the presence of other atherosclerotic aspects such as elevated VLDL and small, dense LDL-C particles. Another explanation is that HDL-C may hinder the development of heart disease by preventing LDL-C oxidation and monocyte binding to arterial cells. In addition, low HDL-C levels commonly are part of the multiple metabolic syndrome. These associations potentially explain why low blood HDL-C is such a powerful risk factor for heart disease and may serve as a marker for the presence of other risk factors.

Lp(a)

Lp(a), the less familiar form of LDL-C, is linked to heart disease and is gaining notoriety among scientists and physicians. Part of the chemical makeup of Lp(a) is similar to that of plasminogen, the clot-dissolving enzyme that binds to the endothelial lining of the arteries. Because of this similarity, Lp(a) interferes with the action of plasminogen, which in turn contributes to blood clot formation and over a prolonged period of time leads to significant arterial wall damage. Blood clots form after plaques rupture, which contributes to heart attacks. Moreover, blood Lp(a) concentrations greater than 25 mg/dL have the same negative effects as LDL-C. Blood Lp(a) is not currently included in the standard cholesterol blood test, though many physicians are adding this measure to their routine screening for heart disease. In addition, the long-term effects of Lp(a)-lowering therapy on the risk of heart disease have not been defined. Therefore, mass Lp(a) screening or interventions directed at lowering blood Lp(a) levels currently is not justified. However, if you have a strong family history of heart disease or if you have coronary artery disease and don't have any of the traditional risk factors, your doctor may advise you to have your Lp(a) level checked. Values above 25 mg/dL are associated with increased risk of heart disease.

If you have elevated Lp(a), it's not clear what you can do about it. Niacin, omega-3 fatty acids, and estrogen may help in some cases. (Talk to your doctor before adding any dietary supplements.) While the effect of Lp(a) on heart disease risk is under further investigation, you should continue to strive for a healthy lifestyle. This includes exercising regularly, controlling weight, and avoiding smoking, as well as eating a diet rich in fruits, vegetables, and whole grains and low in saturated fat and cholesterol.

Postprandial Lipemia

Postprandial lipemia is the time period up to 8 hours following a meal when there is an increase in blood triglycerides. During this time blood triglycerides absorbed through the digestive process quickly rise and then steadily decline. The time it takes after a meal for blood triglyceride levels to return to before-meal levels is generally 6 to 14 hours. Exaggerated or prolonged lipemia (an abnormally long period for triglycerides to return to before-meal levels) is associated with increased heart disease risk. The relationship between postprandial lipemia and heart disease has been established relatively recently in comparison to the relationship between cholesterol and heart disease. Perhaps only in the last 15 years or so have scientists begun to focus on this topic. Both direct and indirect evidence support a relationship between triglyceride-rich lipoproteins and heart disease. A prolonged postprandial lipemia response leads to a number of harmful events associated with arterial plaque buildup. Possibly the most significant finding is the formation of the highly atherosclerotic small, dense LDL-C particles and a reduction in the concentration of protective HDL-C particles. Prolonged postprandial lipemia also enhances thrombosis, or blood clot formation. Genetic makeup affects the magnitude of the postprandial responses, but these responses are also affected by environmental factors such as exercise and diet.

C-Reactive Protein (CRP)

Elevated amounts of C-reactive protein (CRP), a protein found in the blood, are associated with increased risk of heart disease. The reason for the relationship between CRP and heart disease is not completely understood, but CRP is part of the inflammation process and is thought to enhance the removal of unwanted substances from the body. Inflammation occurs with many chronic diseases (e.g., arthritis) as well as injuries (e.g., sprained ankles). When tissue inflammation occurs, the body produces CRP which causes blood CRP levels to increase. Scientists now know that inflammation is part of the heart disease process, and because CRP is associated with inflammation, it is now considered an indicator of heart disease risk. Some scientific information suggests that regular exercise can reduce blood CRP levels.

Summary

Blood lipids and lipoproteins play a major role in the development of heart disease. Elevated total blood cholesterol and LDL-C values are strongly linked to heart disease because both are part of arterial plaque. Oxidized LDL-C, a special form of LDL, promotes SMC growth, enhances platelet adherence to the arterial wall, and impairs normal arterial function. However, a substantial number of heart attacks occur in individuals with only moderate blood cholesterol and LDL-C levels. In these cases, HDL-C values are low and triglycerides are elevated. Thus, having high HDL-C levels seems to protect the heart against disease while elevated triglycerides seem to play a role in encouraging the development of heart disease.

ACTION PLAN:

LINKING CHOLESTEROL AND HEART DISEASE

- ☐ Read about the normal function of the heart and arteries.
- ☐ Be familiar with atherosclerosis and plaque formation, how they inhibit normal artery function, and the primary hypotheses on how and why they develop.
- ☐ Know the risk factors for heart disease and be aware of any that you possess.
- ☐ Learn about the part cholesterol and other lipids and lipoproteins play in the development of heart disease.

CHAPTER 3

EXERCISING TO IMPROVE CHOLESTEROL AND HEALTH

Many Americans do not realize the significant health benefits that are obtained by including physical activity and exercise in their daily routines. While this book focuses on the effects of exercise on cholesterol, there are many other benefits of a regular exercise program. Most important, a physically active lifestyle reduces the risk of dying prematurely from many diseases, including heart disease. Physically active people also are at reduced risk for developing diseases such as colon and breast cancer, diabetes, and the metabolic syndrome. At the same time, a lifestyle that includes physical activity and planned exercise can enhance mental function, promote healthy muscles and bones, help maintain overall body function, and preserve the independence of older adults.

The theoretical relationship among health, fitness, and the quantity of physical activity and exercise necessary for these benefits is presented in figure 3.1. The figure presents two concepts. The first is the relationship between health-related benefits and physical activity, represented by the solid black line. Just a little physical activity and exercise will result in some health-related benefits, while more physical activity and exercise can result in even greater health benefits. The second concept is exercising to increase physical fitness, represented by the dashed line. Exercising at lower intensities (less than 50 percent of maximal functional capacity) has much less effect on fitness than exercising at higher intensities (70 to 80 percent of maximal functional capacity), which results in optimal physical fitness gains as measured by *maximal oxygen consumption.* (We discuss functional capacity later in this chapter.) As a result of planned exercise, you can improve your physical fitness somewhere between 10 to 25 percent. When you incorporate more physical activity or planned

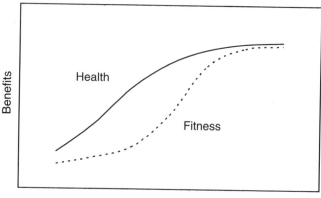

Figure 3.1 Relationship among health, fitness, and quantity of physical activity and exercise necessary for benefits. Small increases in physical activity and exercise can cause significant health benefits, while larger quantities of exercise and physical activity are required for increasing fitness benefits.

Adapted, by permission, from J.L. Durstine, P. Painter, B.A. Franklin, et al, 2000, "Physical activity for the chronically ill and disabled," *Sports Medicine* 30(3): 214.

exercise in your lifestyle and then maintain this activity level throughout your life, the health-related benefits continue to develop.

While the terms *physical activity* and *exercise* are sometimes used interchangeably, there are differences between the two.

- Physical activity is any form of muscular activity that produces contractions of skeletal muscle. Physical activity results in an expenditure of energy proportional to muscular work and is related to health benefits.

- Exercise is a subset of physical activity that consists of planned, structured, and repetitive bodily movement with a goal of improving or maintaining physical fitness. Exercise is defined in terms of frequency, intensity, duration, and specific activities (mode), which is discussed in detail in chapter 5.

These distinctions, while subtle, are important in understanding the role of physical activity and exercise in lowering your cholesterol. In the next section we'll briefly discuss some of the major benefits of an active lifestyle.

Exercising for Health Benefits

More than 60 percent of American adults do not engage in the recommended amount of daily physical activity or planned exercise (DHHS 1996). Women, minority and ethnic groups, the elderly, and children get less physical activity than adult men do. Thus, the American College of Sports Medicine (ACSM) strongly endorses increased lifetime participation in moderate-intensity exercise or physical activity (e.g., brisk walking). This goal enables you to achieve health-related benefits while reducing risk for developing many of the leading causes of premature death, such as cardio-vascular disease, some cancers, and metabolic diseases (ACSM 2005).

Increasing daily physical activity and planned exercise contributes to health in many ways (see the following sidebar). Daily physical activity also increases the body's capacity to do work, which increases the body's ability to meet daily physical needs and the unexpected demands of life and reduces strain to many body systems and organs, including the heart. Also, the more physical activity you complete each day, the greater your daily energy expenditure and health-related benefits. This greater energy expenditure can also assist in weight loss. Increased daily physical activity or planned exercise may in some instances reduce appetite while increasing basal metabolic rate, or the speed at which your body expends energy while at rest. These physiologic changes brought on by increased daily physical activity are in part the reason why exercise is associated with reduced body weight and fat. Reduced body weight and reduced fat are also helpful in reducing blood cholesterol values and in changing the way that cholesterol is carried in the blood.

Benefits of Regular Physical Activity

Regular physical activity performed on most days of the week reduces the risk of developing some of the leading causes of illness and death in the United States. Regular physical activity improves health in the following ways:

- Reduces the risk of dying prematurely
- Reduces the risk of dying from heart disease
- Reduces the risk of developing diabetes
- Reduces the risk of developing high blood pressure
- Reduces blood pressure in people who already have high blood pressure
- Reduces the risk of developing colon cancer
- Reduces feelings of depression and anxiety
- Helps control weight
- Helps build and maintain healthy bones, muscles, and joints
- Helps older adults become stronger and better able to move about without falling
- Promotes psychological well-being

Modified from the US Department of Health and Human Services (US DHHS), 1996, *Physical Activity and Health: A Report of the Surgeon General* (Atlanta: Centers for Disease Control and Prevention, National Center for Chronic Disease Prevention and Health Promotion).

The relationship between physical activity and overall death rates is fairly strong. The more daily physical activity that you complete, the less likely it is that you will die an early death from many diseases. This relationship holds true for most age groups and for various populations from different countries. Furthermore, strong scientific evidence supports even moderate levels of physical activity, such as regular walking, as providing health-related benefits and protection from many diseases. These same health-related benefits are attainable even for adults who adopt a physically active lifestyle later in life.

Exercising to Lower Cholesterol

In the past decade we have gained a much better understanding of blood cholesterol and triglyceride levels and their movement throughout the body as lipoproteins. Currently, we know that many environmental and genetic factors affect lipoprotein movement to various tissues in the body and the amount of blood cholesterol and triglycerides found with the various blood lipoproteins. Factors that affect blood cholesterol, triglyceride, and lipoprotein levels include aging, body fat distribution, dietary composition, cigarette smoking, and regular exercise participation. For example, dietary changes that reduce dietary fat content and increase carbohydrate consumption can positively influence blood cholesterol and the lipoprotein profile, ultimately reducing the risk of heart disease (Durstine et al. 2002).

Regular exercise participation and physical activity also positively affect blood lipid and lipoprotein profiles (see table 3.1). The current scientific understanding is that physical activity or planned exercise positively alters blood triglyceride levels. However, total blood cholesterol is not usually changed after exercise training unless body weight is lowered or dietary composition is changed. What does happen is that the way cholesterol is carried by the blood lipoproteins is changed so that more of the good HDL-C is found in the blood (Durstine et al. 2002).

Attaining Physical Fitness

Physical fitness consists of a set of attributes relating to the body's ability to perform physical activity. Being physically fit means having the strength and endurance to carry out daily activities without undue stress and fatigue, to participate with ample energy in leisure-time pursuits, and to deal with unforeseen emergencies. As you perform more daily physical activity and planned exercise, you become more physically fit. As a result, your heart, lungs, and muscles are stronger while your body

Table 3.1   Effects of Physical Activity and Exercise on Blood Lipids and Lipoproteins

Lipid or lipoprotein	Physical activity and exercise
Triglyceride	Reductions ranging from 4 to 37 percent; average change is approximately 24 percent
Cholesterol	No change unless body weight or diet is altered to reduce consumption of fat
LDL-C	No change unless body weight or diet is altered to reduce consumption of fat
Lp(a)	No change because Lp(a) is genetically determined
HDL-C	Increases ranging from 4 to 22 percent; average change is approximately 8 percent

Adapted, by permission, from J.L. Durstine, P.W. Grandjean, P.G. Davis, et al, 2001, "Blood lipid and lipoprotein adaptations to exercise: A quantitative analysis," *Sports Medicine* 31(15): Appendix I, 1046-1057.

is firmer and more flexible. Your body weight and percentage of body fat are more likely to fall within a desirable range. At the same time, by exercising you lower your risk for various diseases and chronic illnesses (ACSM 2005).

Functional capacity is defined as the body's ability to complete work. The greater your functional capacity, the less fatigue you experience during daily activities. Exercise training increases your functional capacity and is accomplished by increasing cardiovascular endurance, muscular endurance, and muscular strength. Before we discuss these three aspects, note that they are three of five components of physical fitness (the other two components are flexibility and body composition).

Cardiovascular endurance training results in changes in blood lipids and lipoproteins, while resistance exercise training usually results in little or no change. Though the exact reason remains unclear for the lack of lipoprotein change after resistance training, the overall amount of exercise completed, or *calories* burned, during resistance exercise is much smaller than that completed during cardiovascular endurance exercise, which is the likely cause for no change. In some cases, when blood triglyceride levels before exercise training were elevated, resistance training lowered triglyceride levels. Total cholesterol and LDL-C concentrations are only lowered after resistance training when a decrease in body weight or body fat or an increase in lean body mass occurs. HDL-C levels usually are not changed after resistance training, and if increases occur, they are small. In the following section we define the three aspects of fitness in more detail as well as the training they require.

Endurance Exercise

Cardiovascular endurance refers to the heart and the circulation system's ability to complete work over a period of time with little fatigue. Improvement in cardiovascular endurance is achieved through aerobic exercises. Forms of aerobic or endurance exercises include walking, jogging, running, dancing, swimming, bicycling, and many others. Because aerobic or endurance training increases the amount of work that the cardiovascular system can do and also increases the heart's ability to deliver blood and oxygen to the body, it is often referred to as cardiovascular endurance training. In addition to increasing the cardiovascular system's strength and endurance, aerobic exercise also positively affects all the risk factors for heart disease. Because aerobic exercises increase the functional capacity of the cardiovascular system and reduce heart disease risk, they have become the exercise of choice. A certain amount of endurance exercise yields the best health benefits. Read on to find out how much exercise you need for changing your lipid and lipoprotein profile and its effects on each cholesterol component.

Triglycerides

Blood triglyceride values generally decrease after endurance exercise training. These changes are related to the before-exercise values, but more importantly they are related to the volume of exercise completed each week. Individuals with higher triglyceride levels before beginning an exercise program usually experience greater reductions in triglyceride levels after the exercise training intervention is completed. In one exercise study, persons with very high triglyceride levels before starting a physical activity program had tremendous reductions in blood triglyceride values after the program (Kraus et al. 2002). In other studies where blood triglyceride values were in the normal range (around 130 mg/dL before exercise), triglyceride levels were reduced following exercise intervention programs lasting from 3 to 12 months. However, the amount of triglyceride change was not as great as for those individuals with very high before-training values. This information means that endurance exercise decreases blood triglyceride levels in most people but those individuals with the highest initial triglyceride levels receive the greatest reductions and thus the greatest health benefit.

Another concept to remember when considering exercise as a means for reducing blood triglyceride levels is the exercise volume, or the amount of exercise completed during the endurance training program. The greater the volume of exercise you complete, the greater the reduction in blood triglycerides (see figure 3.2), although blood triglyceride levels will never reach a level of zero. For example, a 40-year-old sedentary male, whom we'll call Lyn, completed our heart disease risk factor

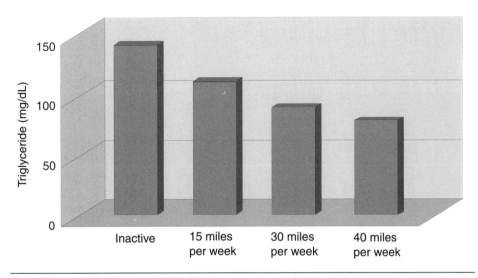

Figure 3.2 Blood triglyceride levels are usually lower in people who are physically active. The more exercise that is completed, the lower the blood triglyceride levels are.

Data from J.L. Durstine, et al., 1987.

screening and exercise testing program, which includes a blood lipid and lipoprotein profile. In Lyn's first blood test his triglyceride levels were approximately 600 mg/dL, four times the amount recommended by the NCEP. After starting an exercise program that began with three exercise sessions (15 minutes per session) per week and progressed to four or five exercise sessions per week (30 minutes per session) over a total of 12 weeks, Lyn's blood triglyceride levels were reduced to 400 mg/dL. This is a good reduction in triglyceride levels, but it is still not near the recommended level. Lyn continued to exercise, and after one year of training five to six days per week for at least 45 minutes per session, his blood triglyceride levels were approximately 250 mg/dL. Lyn was able to bring his blood triglyceride levels close to normal ranges through exercise. However, Lyn responded in the best possible way to exercise training.

One last concept to consider is that blood triglyceride levels are affected almost immediately after starting endurance training. For example, within 10 to 14 days after starting an exercise program consisting of moderate physical activity (brisk walking for 30 minutes four or five days a week), blood triglyceride levels will slowly start to decline. Unfortunately, once regular exercising is stopped, triglyceride levels return to before-exercise levels almost in the same amount of time that it took to reduce them (Gyntelberg et al. 1977). This means you must exercise on a regular basis to maintain the reduction in triglycerides.

Chylomicrons and VLDL.   Blood chylomicrons are the primary carriers of postprandial triglycerides, whereas after a person fasts for a period of 8 or more hours no chylomicrons are found in the blood and VLDL is the primary carrier of blood triglycerides. Because chylomicrons and VLDL are the primary triglyceride carriers and because blood triglyceride levels are reduced after exercise, chylomicrons and VLDL are also lower after exercise. The size of this reduction is directly related to the volume of exercise completed during the endurance exercise program and the initial triglyceride values. In addition to the triglyceride associated with VLDL, a small amount of cholesterol is associated with VLDL, and after an exercise program where VLDL triglyceride is reduced, VLDL-cholesterol is also reduced (Durstine and Thompson 2001).

Postprandial lipemia.   Postprandial lipemia is the period following a meal during which triglyceride levels are elevated over premeal values. Exaggerated postprandial lipemia is when a longer time period is needed to lower blood triglyceride levels following a meal, and it is associated with increased heart disease risk. One of the surest responses to a single exercise session is the reduction of postprandial lipemia. Regular exercise will enhance the results from the single exercise session and further reduce postprandial lipemia for most individuals. Recent research indicates that a reduced postprandial lipemia is associated with reduced heart disease risk (Tjerk et al. 1999).

Cholesterol

Though we often read in newspapers or hear on radio or television reports that exercise lowers blood cholesterol, in general this is not true. Exercise does not necessarily lower blood cholesterol; in fact, most exercise training studies find that blood cholesterol is not altered as a result of exercise training (Durstine et al. 2002). However, under certain conditions blood cholesterol is lower after exercise training. For example, when starting an exercise program, dietary changes are often also made, reducing consumption of dietary fats. This change in conjunction with exercise training can reduce blood cholesterol. A second circumstance is restricting the number of calories consumed when beginning an exercise program and losing body weight as a result; in this case blood cholesterol can also be reduced. For a reduction in blood cholesterol to occur with exercise training, a reduction in dietary fat or body weight must also occur.

Consider again the client Lyn, whom we referred to earlier, and let's examine his other lipid changes. His blood cholesterol at the initial screening and testing period was 214 mg/dL. After the first 12 weeks of exercise his body weight and diet did not change, and his blood cholesterol was 210 mg/dL. However, one year after beginning an exercise program he had lost 30 pounds of weight, stopped smoking, and changed his diet to include less fat. Now his blood cholesterol was 170 mg/dL, and Lyn was

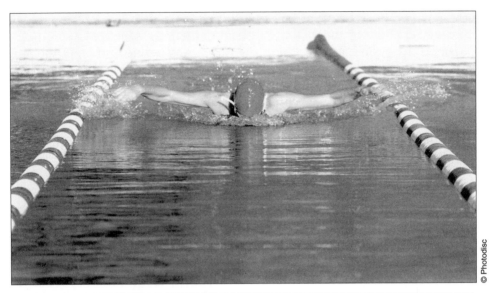

© Photodisc

One of the great things about aerobic exercise, besides its positive effects on cholesterol levels, is the variety of types to choose from.

very conscientious about doing his daily exercise and eating properly. In short, after 12 weeks, though he exercised regularly he did not reduce his body weight or change his diet and his blood cholesterol did not change, whereas for the next nine months he continued to exercise regularly, lost body weight, and altered his diet, resulting in dramatically reduced blood cholesterol levels.

LDL-C

As discussed in chapter 2, LDL-C is the primary means for moving blood cholesterol, and it is elevated in people who eat diets high in fat, especially saturated fats (fats from animal products), or in people who have a genetic tendency for elevated LDL-C. Unfortunately, LDL-C is generally not lower after regular endurance exercise. Although some studies report LDL-C reduction after exercise training, in these cases the subjects reduced dietary fat consumption or decreased their body weight or both (Durstine et al. 2002).

LDL comes in various sizes ranging from smaller, denser LDL particles to larger, less dense particles. The smaller, denser LDL particles are most strongly related to heart disease. Some evidence suggests that regular exercise may reduce the number of small LDL particles, thus reducing overall risk of heart disease. One recent study in healthy but mildly overweight men found that one year after beginning a physical activity program, the number of small LDL particles did change (Kraus et al. 2002). Although the reduction in numbers of small LDL was not statistically significant, both the amount of exercise completed each week and decreased body fat were significantly linked with the reduction in the number of small LDL particles. A second study, evaluating physically active and inactive men with elevated blood cholesterol levels, reported lower blood triglyceride levels and lower numbers of small LDL particles in physically active men (Halle et al. 1997). Certainly, more research is needed in this area, but the early indications are that increased physical activity and reductions in body weight affect the small LDL particles, favoring a reduced risk of heart disease.

Lp(a)

Lp(a) is a form of LDL containing a special protein referred to as apolipoprotein(a). People with Lp(a) levels greater than 25 mg/dL are at extremely high risk for developing premature heart disease. Unfortunately, because Lp(a) is an inherited trait, being physically active or participating in regular exercise does not appear to change blood Lp(a) levels. Medications such as niacin and estrogen are often successful in reducing Lp(a) levels. However, regular exercise participation is still important because you can gain many other potential exercise benefits such as increased functional capacity.

HDL-C

As mentioned in chapter 1, HDL-C is referred to as good cholesterol because it is associated with reduced heart disease risk—elevated blood levels of HDL-C are desired. As is the case with other lipoproteins, HDL-C is affected by genetics as well as environmental factors. Factors improving HDL-C levels include exercise, reductions in some dietary influences, body weight reduction, and body composition change. HDL-C is generally responsive to endurance exercise training and it increases in a dose-dependent manner (see figure 3.3). This means that the more you exercise the more HDL-C increases. Still, exercise programs must last at least 12 weeks to increase HDL-C values. These exercise-induced HDL-C increases usually range from 4 to 22 percent while the actual values range from 2 mg/dL to 8 mg/dL. In individuals whose genetics make them less likely to respond, endurance exercise may not result in an increased blood HDL-C level (Durstine et al. 2001).

The length of the exercise training and the amount of exercise completed each week has an important role in determining HDL-C change. Twelve weeks of exercise training usually increases blood HDL-C values. However, when the program length is shorter than 12 weeks, blood HDL-C changes are not likely. Perhaps the most important consideration for HDL-C change after exercise training is the amount of exercise completed.

Percentage body fat is another factor involved with exercise-induced HDL-C change after exercise. Reductions in body fat are associated with

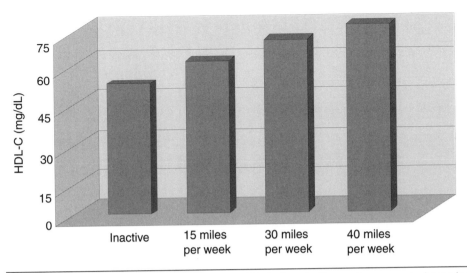

Figure 3.3 The exercise-induced increase in HDL-C rises further as the amount of exercise increases.

Data from J.L. Durstine, et al., 1987.

elevations in HDL-C. In science, this is referred to as an inverse relationship because one factor goes down, in this case body fat, and another factor goes up, in this case HDL-C. Weight loss associated with caloric restriction or caloric restriction and exercise that causes reductions in percentage of body fat is also linked with increased HDL-C values. Most important, when calorie-restricted diets are combined with exercise, greater changes in body composition and HDL-C are found. Exercise-induced HDL-C increases are found both in the presence and absence of reduced body fat, and exercise training without altered body weight or composition can increase HDL-C, but this increase is further enhanced if body fat is reduced.

Much like LDL, HDL particles come in various sizes ranging from smaller, denser particles to larger, less dense particles. These larger particles are referred to as HDL_2 particles. Unlike the small LDL, which is strongly related to an increased risk of heart disease, the larger, less dense HDL_2 particles are inversely related to heart disease risk, meaning the more particles there are, the lower the risk of heart disease. Exercise training generally results in higher HDL_2.

Let's return to Lyn. His initial blood HDL-C level was 38 mg/dL before he started exercising regularly, which was below the NCEP recommendation of 40 mg/dL. After 12 weeks of exercise, his HDL-C level was 41 mg/dL. Over a year he increased his exercise training, changed his diet, lost weight, reduced his body fat, and stopped smoking. These were all the right changes and as a result he was able to optimize his blood lipid and lipoprotein levels. Lyn's HDL-C was 46 mg/dL (a 15 percent increase), and he became a success story.

Several benefits are attributed to regular exercise. A single exercise session may raise HDL-C and HDL_2-C during the 24- to 48-hour period after exercise. Knowing this fact and the fact that exercise training can also increase HDL-C, we can state with confidence that both a single exercise session and regular exercise training have positive and independent effects on the blood lipid and lipoprotein profiles. This information supports the notion that exercise should be performed at least every other day to maximize its benefits.

Resistance Exercise

Aerobic fitness is best enhanced by cardiovascular exercise training, while muscular fitness is best enhanced by weight or resistance training. Muscular fitness has two components, endurance and strength. When developing a complete fitness program, you should include muscular endurance and strength exercises. Weight or resistance exercise is usually completed two or three days per week and involves completing one to three circuits (one circuit consists of 5 to 8 exercise stations), performing 6 to 14 repetitions per station, and resting briefly between stations (20 seconds to 2 minutes). Resistance training of this type is usually completed in 30 to 40 minutes.

Muscular endurance is the ability of a specific skeletal muscle group to sustain work over a period of time. Acquiring muscular endurance is specific to the muscle groups involved, meaning that if you work your arms, your arms develop muscular endurance, not your legs. In order to improve both arm and leg endurance, you would need to do exercises that involve both arms and legs. The overall goal of a muscular endurance program is to increase the amount of time until your muscles become fatigued. In order to achieve this goal, lighter weights with many repetitions are used. You should incorporate physical activities into your lifestyle that require muscular endurance. As you progress in your program and your endurance improves, you should add small amounts of weight. With greater muscular endurance, you are less likely to develop muscle fatigue.

Muscular strength is the muscle's ability to produce maximal force against resistance during one contraction. The stronger you are, the greater the force you can produce in one effort. In contrast to muscular endurance, the focus of this type of resistance training is to complete fewer repetitions with greater amounts of weight. As you progress in your resistance training and as your strength increases, you should continually add additional resistance or weight. In addition, you may increase the frequency of your training sessions and add additional exercise sets to elicit greater strength gains.

Resistance exercise usually does not result in the same lipid and lipoprotein changes as endurance exercise. We do not completely understand why little change occurs—but the reason is likely related to the smaller volume of exercise completed in resistance training. Resistance exercise does not alter blood triglyceride levels even when initial levels are high. Total blood cholesterol and LDL-C values are also unchanged after resistance training. However, as is the case with endurance exercise training, decreases in levels of small blood cholesterol and LDL-C are found with resistance training when percentage body fat is decreased and lean body mass is increased. Still, when total body mass, lean body mass, and percentage body fat are unchanged, cholesterol and LDL-C remain unchanged.

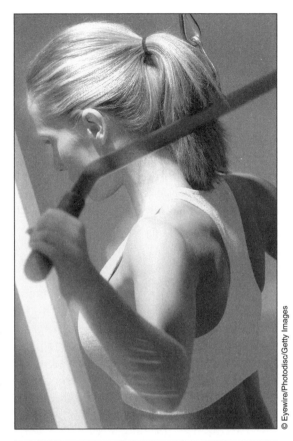

Strength training enhances a regular aerobic fitness program and yields overall health benefits.

HDL-C changes after resistance training are not found. Collectively, no consistent link exists between resistance exercise and cholesterol and lipoprotein changes. Even though resistance exercise may not affect blood cholesterol and the cholesterol associated with the lipoproteins, the benefits of muscular endurance and strength that result are still important in developing overall health and fitness.

Body Composition and Flexibility

As mentioned, body composition and flexibility are the two other components of physical fitness in addition to aerobic fitness and muscular strength and endurance. Body composition refers to the percentage of body weight that is fat tissue and the percentage that is fat-free, or lean, tissue. Excess body fat is associated with hypertension, type 2 diabetes, and hyperlipidemia. Generally, a benefit of being physically active is a reduction in body fat and an increase in lean tissue. This in turn has a positive effect on the blood cholesterol and lipoprotein profile, hypertension, and type 2 diabetes.

Flexibility refers to the ability of a joint to move through a complete range of motion. Though flexibility is important in athletic performance, it is also essential for carrying out daily activities. Flexibility depends on many conditions, including the joint's ability to stretch, the compliance (tightness) of tissue such as ligaments and tendons, and adequate warm-up. Also, just as muscular strength is specific to the muscle groups involved, flexibility is joint-specific. Because of this joint-specific characteristic, you will need to include flexibility exercises that involve all joints in the body. When you incorporate flexibility exercises (also called stretching and range-of-motion exercises) into an exercise program, your flexibility increases.

Physical Activity

Physical activity and planned exercise should be part of every person's lifestyle. Throughout this chapter we have talked about the benefits of exercise training on the cholesterol and lipoprotein profile. In this section we focus on the effects of being physically active on the cholesterol and lipoprotein profile. First, physical activity is not necessarily planned exercise (see the discussion of the differences between the two on page 30). The physical activity that is part of your everyday activities can provide many health benefits. The more physical activity in your daily life, the greater the health benefits you receive. For example, climbing the stairs instead of riding the elevator is one way of incorporating more physical activity into your daily routine. Another example is parking your car farther away from where you are going. As a result of climbing the stairs and walking greater distances, you add more physical activity to your lifestyle, and this increased daily activity results in health benefits.

About 50 years ago a researcher named Dr. Jeremy Morris evaluated London bus drivers and ticket takers. Bus drivers sit most of the day while the ticket takers walk up and down the aisles and climb the stairs of the double-deck buses as they collect tickets. Dr. Morris found that the drivers had more health problems, including heart disease, than did ticket takers (Morris et al. 1966). Many of the increased medical problems were attributed to the job inactivity of the drivers. The drivers were more likely to have high blood pressure, be obese, and have abnormal blood lipid profiles. Thus, physical activity influences the blood lipid profile, but the question is, how much activity is necessary to effect a change?

Optimizing Exercise to Improve Cholesterol

About 1,200 to 1,500 kcals of energy expenditure each week is needed to optimize your blood lipid and lipoprotein profile (Durstine et al. 2001). This is equal to a brisk walk or slow jog for approximately two to three miles six days each week. Though this seems a straight answer, there are other considerations. For one, different levels or thresholds of energy expenditure exist for causing lipid and lipoprotein changes. For example, a sedentary person who starts a daily exercise program can expect to see a reduction in blood triglycerides within several weeks. The amount of energy expenditure or the volume of exercise necessary for triglyceride change is lower than that required for other lipid changes. HDL-C changes, on the other hand, take several months of regular exercise and weekly expenditures of 1,200 to 1,500 kcal.

Another point to consider is your state of training. If you are physically inactive, becoming physically active will cause some blood lipid and lipoprotein change, but if you are already physically active or follow a planned exercise program and have elevated HDL-C levels, you will need to incorporate more physical activity and planned exercise in order to get additional lipid and lipoprotein changes. Integrating as much physical activity as possible into your lifestyle is important, but in order to optimize blood lipid and lipoprotein changes, you need to include planned exercise in your daily routine.

The more you exercise, the greater the lipid and lipoprotein changes you are likely to achieve. However, once you have achieved 1,200 to 1,500 kcal of weekly energy expenditure, you will need to exercise more to achieve greater lipid and lipoprotein changes. At some level, greater amounts of exercise will provide fewer changes. This means that you need greater increases in exercise to get greater blood lipid and lipoprotein changes. For many people, 1,200 to 1,500 kcal of energy expenditure each week is a reachable goal.

A final point for consideration is the possibility of dividing exercise into more than one daily session. If, for example, your plan incorporates 30 minutes of daily exercise, you can get roughly the same improvements in your blood lipid and lipoprotein profile by doing multiple daily exercise sessions that total 30 minutes. Several studies have evaluated the benefits of multiple exercise sessions in one day that add up to the same total exercise time and energy expenditure as that in a single session (e.g., two 15-minute exercise sessions that total 30 minutes). Results from these studies suggest that exercising for 30 minutes in one daily exercise session provides the same lipid and lipoprotein profile benefit as exercising for two 15-minute exercise sessions in one day (Donnelly et al. 2000).

Many people aren't sure whether walking or jogging is the best type, or mode, of exercise to get the greatest lipid and lipoprotein change. The answer is easy: You can get the same lipid and lipoprotein change regardless of the mode of exercise you choose, and there are many exercises, such as bike riding, rowing, and hiking, to choose from. Your goal is to expend energy equal to 1,200 to 1,500 kcal per week. The mode of exercise is not as important as reaching this required energy expenditure. Chapter 5 gives more information on how to determine if you're expending 1,200 to 1,500 kcal per week.

The intensity of the exercise session, or how hard you work, is important. However, although exercise intensity has some role in optimizing lipid and lipoprotein changes, the most important consideration is the volume of exercise completed. You can argue that the faster and harder you work, the greater the volume of exercise you complete in a set time period. Unfortunately, this argument is not always correct. If the exercise intensity is too high, you may not be able to exercise long enough to reach the required volume of exercise necessary to optimize your blood lipid and lipoprotein profile. The appropriate exercise intensity ranges from 40 to 60 percent of your maximal exercise level; it is the work rate achieved by brisk walking or slow jogging for at least 30 minutes. Chapter 5 will detail how to calculate your maximal exercise level and how to measure exercise intensity.

Finally, some people's bodies will respond to increased physical activity and planned exercise programming by improving the blood lipid and lipoprotein profile, but some will not. Many factors contribute to your lipid and lipoprotein profile, and one of these factors is genetics. There is evidence that most people respond to exercise, or are *responders,* while the few individuals who do not respond to exercise or respond with less than optimal lipid and lipoprotein changes are referred to as *nonresponders.* The lipoprotein Lp(a) is a good example. Exercise does not effect a change in this lipoprotein because it is genetically determined.

Summary

In this chapter you have learned that incorporating both physical activity and planned exercise will result in many health benefits, including lower risk for certain diseases. We have discussed the importance and benefits of a lifestyle that includes both physical activity and planned exercise in order to optimize the lipid and lipoprotein profile. We also reviewed the concept of thresholds of energy expenditure and the need to meet these thresholds in order to increase the likelihood of changing blood lipids and lipoproteins. Daily exercise of 15 to 20 minutes will result in minimal blood triglyceride change and most likely little or no HDL-C change, whereas daily planned exercise performed at a moderate intensity, such as a brisk walk or slow jog that can be maintained for 30 minutes or more, with an overall exercise program that lasts for at least 12 weeks, is necessary to change HDL-C levels. These 30 minutes of moderate exercise may be performed in one daily session or may be split into multiple exercise sessions, such as two 15-minute periods.

ACTION PLAN:

EXERCISING TO IMPROVE CHOLESTEROL AND HEALTH

☐ Take stock of the many health benefits available through regular physical activity and exercise.

☐ Understand that the amount of exercise that will yield general health benefits is less than the amount needed to increase physical fitness.

☐ Note the importance of exercise to change the way cholesterol is carried in the body, especially its help in increasing HDL-C levels.

☐ Learn how cholesterol is affected by each component of physical fitness:

- Cardiovascular fitness
- Muscular strength
- Muscular endurance
- Flexibility
- Body composition

☐ Know the amount of weekly energy expenditure needed to optimize your cholesterol profile and the factors that go into determining this amount.

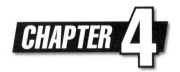

CHAPTER 4

SETTING GOALS TO MODIFY CHOLESTEROL

I n the first chapters of this book you learned that blood cholesterol is involved in many bodily functions, but when it is elevated, you are at risk for developing several diseases, specifically heart disease. You also learned where blood cholesterol comes from, how it is carried in the blood as lipoproteins, the effects of physical activity and planned exercise on blood cholesterol, and the overall health-related benefits you gain from a lifestyle that includes moderate levels of daily physical activity and planned exercise. The remaining chapters focus on four interventions that can positively alter blood cholesterol and the way cholesterol is carried in the blood (see the following sidebar for an overview of this comprehensive approach to managing blood cholesterol). This chapter prepares you to start changing your lifestyle so that you can reduce your blood cholesterol, optimize your daily physical activity and planned exercise, and reduce your overall risk for premature heart disease.

Comprehensive Approach to Controlling Blood Cholesterol

Blood cholesterol is affected by many factors, including genetics, diet, exercise, and medications. Because many factors can cause elevated blood cholesterol, you should talk to your physician about the proper approach for you to take to reduce your blood cholesterol. A comprehensive approach to lowering blood cholesterol includes making dietary changes such as reducing consumption of dietary fat and cholesterol, beginning an exercise program, and (when necessary) taking medications. For further information, see the NCEP Web site (www.nhlbi.nih.gov/about/ncep/index.htm).

Making Successful Lifestyle Changes

Like most people, you've probably made New Year's resolutions to quit smoking, lose weight, or begin exercising, and perhaps you have even stuck with such resolutions for a while. Too often, however, life gets in the way, and we watch our best intentions fall by the wayside. For most people, making lifestyle changes is not easy. Maintaining change is even harder when you want to make more than one change at once. Scientists have identified five stages of change that most people go through along the way to adopting new behaviors. Being aware of these stages can help you make lifestyle changes. Also know that you can begin making a change at any of these points. Figure 4.1 leads you through a step-by-step method of determining your stage.

- Precontemplation—Not even thinking about change.
- Contemplation—Giving change a thought now and then, but not acting on it.
- Preparation—Doing the new behavior irregularly.
- Action—Doing the new behavior consistently but for less than six months.
- Maintenance—Maintaining the new behavior for six months or more.

Precontemplation is that stage of the change process where you have not developed a desire to change your behavior in the next six months. A six-month period is used because most people need this amount of time to plan a specific behavior change. People in this stage may even lack awareness about specific behaviors they need to change. On the other hand, some people in this stage are very aware of the consequences of their behavior but they avoid making a change because they have not felt the consequences of not doing so. Finally, you may have tried but failed to make the change and have moved on without making the change.

One way to aid in making the move from the precontemplation stage to the contemplation stage is to increase your awareness of the need for the change. Many different avenues exist for increasing awareness, but mass media is by far the largest influence for increasing awareness. In the contemplation stage you intend to change a behavior within the next six months. Like the precontemplation stage, the contemplation stage can last about six months. In this stage you are likely aware of the benefits of the behavior change as well as some of the barriers for achieving the desired behavior. Now you should develop a plan for making your change. The first part of this plan is to set both short-term and long-term goals. Short-term goals should be reasonable and attainable, because the achievement of short-term goals helps ensure successful behavior change by increasing

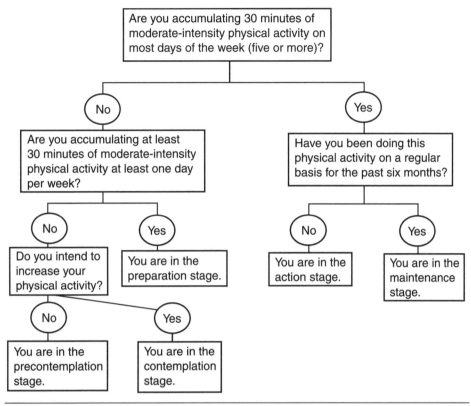

Figure 4.1 Schematic representation of readiness for behavior change. The questions in this figure can help you gauge how ready you are to change. Knowing your stage can help you discover what you need to do to move forward.

Adapted, by permission, from A.V. Carron, P.A. Estabrooks, and H.A. Hausenblas, 2003, *The psychology of physical activity* (New York, NY: McGraw-Hill Higher Education), 159-170.

self-efficacy and developing your confidence for making desired behavior changes.

Barriers provide reasons for not making a change. They are different for each person, and you need to overcome them in order to make a change. Examples of barriers include the finances associated with making the behavior change, family problems that prohibit the change, and a lack of desire to make the change.

If you face these sorts of barriers, you may need extra help to successfully achieve change. In this case, you should seek encouragement and motivation from others in order to move into the next stage. A health-promotion professional has the ability to help you manipulate your environment so you can make the desired behavior change.

Seeking help from others is an indication that you are ready to go beyond the contemplation stage into the preparation stage. The preparation stage is when you intend to make a change within the next 30 days and have already attempted at least once to make this specific change. It is in this stage that you are most likely to have success in making a change.

The action stage is the time up to six months after the preparation stage. It is where you are most likely to make a sufficient behavior change and reflects consistent, positive performance of a desired behavior pattern. You can usually measure the amount of change you've made by determining or measuring the behavior change. For example, if the behavior change is to abstain from drug use or cigarette smoking, you can determine success by measuring the length of time you've abstained from drug use or smoking. In the case of lowering blood cholesterol, success is having lower blood cholesterol after intervention. If your behavior change is to start an exercise program, a means for determining success is the number of times each week that you exercise. After performing the behavior regularly for six months, you are ready to move into the fifth stage, maintenance.

The maintenance stage can last for several years, hopefully for a lifetime. The behavior being changed is the key factor in determining how long this stage lasts. Once you've developed a lifestyle that will lower your blood cholesterol, you need to maintain this lifestyle for the rest of your life.

Preventing Relapses

Relapses can happen at any time. You will need to learn to anticipate and cope with problems associated with falling back into old behavior patterns. Relapses are probably the biggest challenge you will face as you change your eating habits and begin an exercise program. You can help yourself prepare for relapses by knowing that they can happen and that you will have to find ways to reduce the likelihood for relapse.

Behavior change takes place in stages, and progress isn't always in the desired direction. Many times for every two steps forward there may be one step back. That's normal. Every move, forward or back, is part of the overall process of change. You may stay in one stage for a long time before you move forward, or you may go through another stage quickly, stay in that stage for a short time, stumble, and go back to an earlier stage for a while. This isn't a sign of failure. Rather, it's a sign that you're trying to make a change.

The key to successful change is using techniques such as keeping track of your progress, recruiting help from friends or professionals, and thinking positively. These techniques are very helpful in overcoming barriers and preventing lapses. In the following material, we consider each of these techniques separately.

One important technique that you can easily do is keep track of your progress and what you do in your program for change. Most people use some form of diary or log. For example, for an exercise program, items for the log could include the date, time of day, what your activity was, how much time you spent doing the activity, and, if appropriate, the distance traveled (e.g., walked two miles in 30 minutes, ran three miles in 35 minutes, attended a spinning class for 45 minutes). You may want to include other items like how you felt and what your heart rates were.

Another strategy that many exercisers find helpful is teaming up with a friend. Most people like the idea of exercising with a buddy. This technique requires you to report to another person, which can encourage you to continue in an exercise program. Having someone to talk with while you exercise can also make the time go faster.

Another idea that can aid you in making change is obtaining help from a professional trainer. Having a paid personal trainer, especially at the start of an exercise program, will get you started doing the right exercises with the correct forms. A trainer will also encourage and aid you in overcoming barriers to regular participation in an exercise program.

One last technique that you must use is being positive toward exercise. For some people this may not be a problem, but many others would rather take medicine than exercise. Currently, there simply is not a medicine that will give you the benefits of exercise that were discussed in chapter 3. Very little expense is associated with starting and maintaining an exercise program, whereas medicine can be expensive. In maintaining a positive attitude toward regular exercise, I like to think of exercise as a medicine. I often joke with my friends about taking my medicine today—meaning that I exercised. Part of developing a positive outlook toward exercise is knowing that every time you exercise, you are providing yourself with many health-related benefits.

Scientific studies show that these techniques can help reduce the potential for relapse. The principles that are emphasized in the remainder of this chapter are designed to help you

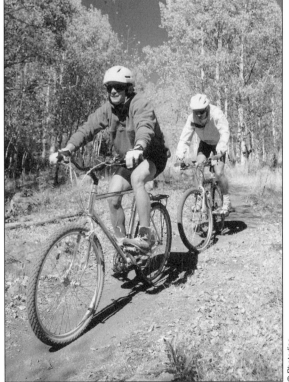

© Photodisc

Exercising with a friend and participating in those activities you truly enjoy are two strategies to increase motivation and help you meet your exercise goals.

succeed in lowering your blood cholesterol, developing a physical activity program, and starting and maintaining a planned exercise program. Small changes are the first step toward long-term change and improving your health, and the best way to improve your health is to develop behaviors associated with a healthy lifestyle.

Overcoming Barriers to Change

Everyone has his or her own personal barriers to change. However, there are several ways to get past these barriers and make lifestyle changes. One important way to overcome a barrier is to simply know that you can reduce your risk for heart disease by lowering your blood cholesterol level. Knowledge is a strong motivational tool for making behavioral changes. The remainder of this book will give you many other ways to help you reach your goals. Hopefully you have already found some of your own reasons to motivate you to find ways to overcome your barriers. Each of us has one or two reasons that are especially important and are powerful enough to get us going even when we're not in the mood. You need to find what these reasons are for you.

Many environmental and personal factors can help you overcome barriers for making change. The following material should give greater insight into what these factors are and how you can use them. The first factor is reinforcement, which can be either a positive or negative consequence of behavior. Positive reinforcement is a reward that you gain as a result of making progress toward a goal, whereas negative reinforcement is a negative consequence to help you get moving in the right direction. For example, if your goal is to lower your blood cholesterol and you succeed, a positive reinforcement is a reward, like a new piece of clothing. On the other hand, if your blood cholesterol stays the same or gets higher, a negative reinforcement is making some kind of compensation, for example, paying a fine or giving up a special activity until you make progress in the correct direction. Most people prefer to use positive reinforcement rather than negative reinforcement because they would rather get a reward than give up an activity they like.

In addition to understanding the importance of reinforcement, you should be aware that you may have limits for changing your blood cholesterol levels. Everyone can change their blood cholesterol by using any of the interventions described in the remainder of this book (e.g., exercise and nutrition). The question is how much can your levels change? Every person has a genetically determined capacity for changing their blood cholesterol. Even though genetics is a powerful factor in regulating blood cholesterol, you can expect a blood cholesterol change of approximately 25 percent or more as a result of good nutrition, physical activity, and planned exercise.

To facilitate change you must not only believe that you can make the change happen, you must work at making the change. Because your blood cholesterol is dependent on many factors, you will need to focus on more than one of these factors. Successful change only comes by following recommendations for developing good nutritional habits, adding daily physical activity to your lifestyle, and setting aside time each day for exercising.

Another point to consider when making lifestyle changes is that behavior can be influenced by personal beliefs and feelings as well as the surrounding environment. If, for example, you have strong feelings about your appearance in exercise clothing, this is a barrier to your exercising, and you will need to develop a plan for overcoming this obstacle. In this case you could wear exercise clothing that solves your concerns about your appearance. The purchase of new clothes for some people is positive reinforcement for exercising. Another consideration is your environment, which includes being around people who want to achieve similar goals as you. Ways to improve your environment include getting an exercise buddy, joining an exercise group, or hiring a personal trainer.

When evaluating whether a cholesterol-reduction program is successful, you only need to answer the following question: Did you lower your blood cholesterol? If the answer to the question is yes, then the intervention was successful. Reducing blood cholesterol is a complex process because blood cholesterol is affected by so many factors, but you have several intervention options to choose from, including starting a planned exercise program and altering your diet. This is the time to consider setting some goals.

Setting Goals

Goal setting is a powerful technique that can help you develop proper blood cholesterol levels. At its simplest, the goal-setting process allows you to choose the interventions you want to use to lower your blood cholesterol. By knowing precisely what you want to achieve and setting proper goals, you are more likely to achieve your goal. Goal setting can give you long-term vision and short-term motivation, all while helping you focus on lowering your blood cholesterol. By setting sharp, clearly defined, realistic goals, you can easily measure success by reaching that goal, and in addition you can take pride in the achievement.

The way in which you set goals strongly influences their effectiveness. When beginning the goal-setting process, keep the SMART (specific, measurable, attainable, realistic, and time-oriented) principle in mind.

Specific. People who set specific goals are more likely to achieve those goals. For example, in developing an exercise program you might set a goal of walking for 15 minutes each morning rather than simply stating,

"I'll exercise more this week." Another example of a specific goal might be to lower your blood cholesterol level to 200 mg/dL in six months.

Measurable.   Exercising more is a commendable idea, but it's not a measurable goal. Walking five miles three days a week is a measurable goal. You should set goals that are measurable and fall within a specific time frame. For example, lowering your blood cholesterol by 15 mg/dL in four weeks is a measurable goal (15 mg/dL) in a specific time period (four weeks).

Attainable.   Setting goals is a skill you acquire through practice. You should set goals so that they are slightly out of your immediate grasp but not so far out of your reach that you have no hope of achieving them. No one will put serious effort into achieving a goal that seems unattainable. Believing that a goal is unattainable also hinders you from ever reaching that goal. As you set goals, try to determine whether they are attainable under your present circumstances. Account for concerns such as being tired, needing rest, and being overcommitted. Develop goals to meet programming recommendations, but feel free to adjust these goals as your personal factors change. Review your goals once again to assure yourself that they are attainable.

Realistic.   Are you one of those people who always expect their best performance? Setting goals for best performance, whatever best performance means, is not always realistic. Unrealistic expectations ignore the inevitable backsliding that occurs and the many factors that aid you in getting to your specific goal. You are better off setting goals that raise your average performance and enhance your progress toward meeting those goals more consistently. For example, you might set a long-term goal to reduce your blood cholesterol to 200 mg/dL in six months.

Time-oriented.   Short-term goals are useful in helping you go the distance in achieving goals. If your long-term goal is to lower your blood cholesterol below 200 mg/dL in two months, you may not reach that goal in that short time period. A different approach would be to set several short-term goals to modify your diet to include less fat and to reduce your body weight by five to eight pounds in two months. Also remember that lower blood cholesterol depends on several considerations, including your initial blood cholesterol levels and your genetic potential for elevated blood cholesterol. If your blood cholesterol is very high, you may have to develop several short-term goals to better enable you to reach your long-term goal. Another example of setting short-term goals involves exercise programming. If your goal is to walk an hour a day, five days a week, you may want to set several short-term goals leading up to this long-term goal. A good short-term goal might be to walk for two 15-minute sessions on Tuesday, Thursday, and Saturday. Then gradually increase the number of minutes you spend and the number of days a week you walk until you reach your long-term goal. In the previous paragraph we mentioned reducing blood cholesterol to 200 mg/dL in six months as an example of a realistic long-term goal. Setting a short-term goal to reduce your blood cholesterol by 15 mg/dL in the next four weeks is a useful way to help reach your long-term goal.

The following sidebar gives a few more suggestions on setting goals, measuring success, and evaluating the next step for those goals. A sample goal-recording sheet is also provided.

Recording, Measuring, and Evaluating Goals

Use the form in figure 4.2 to set your goals. Goals should be specific, measurable, attainable, realistic, and time-oriented. An example of a long-term goal is to lower blood cholesterol below 200 mg/dL in the next six months. This goal is specific, realistic, and has a time frame. After setting long-term goals, you also need to set short-term goals. An example of a short-term goal is to follow the NCEP guidelines and seek professional help in the next two weeks to develop a nutritious diet for reducing body weight in order to lower your blood cholesterol. Evaluation of progress toward this goal is easy: Did you seek help in the two-week time period? After seeking professional dietary help, the next short-term goal is to follow the prescribed diet for at least eight weeks. Evaluation of this short-term goal would include a positive response to the following question: After eight weeks did you follow the diet, lose body weight, and reduce your blood cholesterol? You are now ready to develop your next short-term goal in your journey to reduce your blood cholesterol.

▷ Developing Goals

My long-term goal is _____

_____

I plan to achieve this goal by_____ (date).

My short-term goal is _____

_____

I plan to achieve this goal by_____ (date).

I plan to monitor or measure my progress toward each short- and long-term goal by doing the following: _____

_____

_____

_____

Figure 4.2 Sample worksheet for goals.

From *Action Plan for High Cholesterol* by J. Larry Durstine, 2006, Champaign, IL: Human Kinetics.

Another example of a long-term goal is exercising 30 minutes to one hour every day for at least five days a week within the next six months. A first short-term goal is to walk for 15 minutes Tuesday, Thursday, and Saturday for the next three weeks. After the three-week period, you should evaluate your progress toward this short-term goal. This evaluation is easily done if your answer is yes to the following question: Are you walking for 15 minutes, three days a week? Now you are ready to develop your next short-term goal. When you meet each short-term goal, you should establish a new set of short-term goals that is in line with each long-term goal.

Recognizing the Power of Feedback

When you achieve a goal, take the time to enjoy the satisfaction of achievement. Absorb the implications of the achievement, and observe the progress you have made toward other goals. If the goal was a significant one or one that you had worked toward for some time, take the opportunity to reward yourself appropriately. I might reward myself with a new exercise outfit, a weekend at the beach, or an afternoon at a local air show. Figure out what your rewards are and work toward getting them.

Feedback when you have failed to reach a goal can come from yourself or others. In the quest to lower your blood cholesterol, you may fail to reach a short-term goal of reducing your blood cholesterol by 15 mg/dL in four weeks. Such setbacks happen, but you must learn from your mistakes. Reasons for failure include not trying hard enough, not following the dietary or exercise recommendations, lacking skills or knowledge about dietary or exercise instructions, and setting unrealistic goals. When you fail, ask yourself, "How can I use this information to readjust my goal so that I can succeed?" Using feedback in this fashion can turn failures into positive learning experiences—even failing to meet a goal is a step toward finding a way to succeed if you use the information correctly! The fact that you are trying to change, even if you fail, often opens doors that would otherwise have remained closed, and when used properly, failure can lead to success.

Feedback when you succeed in achieving a goal is a powerful tool for setting and achieving your next goals. First, as we have already mentioned, you need to provide yourself with a reward for achieving a goal. You deserve that reward, so do not skip past it. Here are some other ideas to keep in mind as you develop your new goals for lowering your blood cholesterol.

- If the previous goal was easily achieved, make your next goal harder.
- If the goal took a dispiriting amount of time to achieve, make the next goal a little easier.

- If you learned something that would lead you to change goals that are still outstanding, do so.

Goals change as time moves on, and you should adjust your goals regularly to reflect this personal growth. If goals no longer hold any attraction, let them go. Goal setting is your servant, not your master, and it should bring you pleasure, satisfaction, and a sense of achievement.

Summary

The key to successful movement through the five stages for behavior change is using the techniques described in this chapter. Some of these techniques and strategies include recruiting help from friends or professionals such as personal trainers, overcoming barriers, preventing lapses, thinking positively, and using failure to set new goals. The principles presented in this chapter should have helped you learn useful ways to lower your blood cholesterol and develop a physical activity or planned exercise program. The best way to improve your health is to develop behaviors associated with a healthy lifestyle, and small changes are the first steps toward the overall behavior change and improving your life.

ACTION PLAN:
SETTING GOALS TO MODIFY CHOLESTEROL

☐ Determine your stage of readiness to change, which ranges from just starting to think about it to a solid grounding in the habit.

☐ Identify barriers you face and develop strategies to avoid or overcome these barriers.

☐ Set goals for your exercise and eating plans and your cholesterol profile, making sure they are specific, measurable, attainable, realistic, and time-oriented.

☐ Use feedback to motivate yourself and determine when changes to your goals or program are needed.

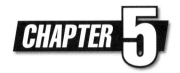

CHAPTER 5

BUILDING AN EXERCISE PROGRAM

Gaining health benefits while reducing risk of heart disease can be accomplished by increasing the amount of physical activity in your lifestyle and by developing a planned exercise program to increase your physical fitness. In this chapter, you will learn concepts that can help you incorporate more physical activity into your lifestyle and principles that are essential for developing a planned exercise program. You can use this information to tailor a physical activity program or planned exercise program to meet your specific needs. This program is one that you will find not too time-consuming yet can help you derive health benefits.

When considering making these behavior changes, it's perfectly normal to have lots of questions about physical activity and planned exercise. What's the best physical activity or exercise to participate in? How do you get the most out of more daily physical activity or planned exercise? How long should exercise sessions last? When developing an exercise program, should you emphasize both cardiovascular endurance *(aerobic fitness)* and muscular strength and endurance *(anaerobic fitness)*? Perhaps the most important question to ask is, How much daily physical activity and planned exercise is necessary to cause a change in blood lipids and lipoproteins? Such questions about physical activity and planned exercise are addressed in this chapter.

We'll start by answering the last question first: How much daily physical activity or planned exercise do you need to positively alter your blood lipid and lipoprotein profile? Generally speaking, the scientific literature indicates that the total volume of physical activity and planned exercise that you need to complete each week is 1,200 to 1,500 kcal of energy expenditure, or 250 kcal per day (roughly 30 to 45 minutes of physical activity and planned exercise).

Setting Long-Term Goals

Using the information from the last chapter, you should set a long-term goal for adding more physical activity and planned exercise into your daily routine in the next two weeks. Make your goal specific, measurable, attainable, and realistic. Using these guides, you can set an appropriate goal and incorporate more daily physical activity and planned exercise into your lifestyle, but before setting your first physical activity goal, realize that there are numerous ways to achieve this goal without making a huge time commitment.

As previously discussed, to change your blood lipid and lipoprotein levels you will need to increase your daily physical activity and planned exercise to approximately 250 kcal of energy expenditure each day or 45 minutes each day. This translates to about four or five hours of total activity each week. Don't let the idea of this amount of time trouble you, because you will start off slowly with a time commitment of less than one or two hours a week. Over the next year, this time commitment will increase to four or five hours.

Your overall long-term goal is to increase your daily physical activity and planned exercise program, such as in the following goal:

> Your long-term goal is to increase the amount of time for your daily physical activity and planned exercise to four to five hours each week by the end of the next 12 months (about 45 minutes each day), expending about 250 kcal each day.

Next, you should set short-term goals that you can modify in order to reach this long-term goal, as we will discuss in the next section.

Adding Physical Activity

A variety of physical activities are suitable for modifying blood cholesterol and lipoprotein levels. They include walking, playing outdoor games with your children or grandchildren, walking the dog, mowing the lawn, doing leisure activities such as gardening or carpentry work, and using the stairs in your office or apartment building rather than using the elevator.

Developing an active lifestyle means finding time in your day for these activities, but don't let time be a barrier. Incorporating more walking into your daily routine can easily be accomplished without requiring much additional time. For example, you can park your car farther away from the building where you work and walk the additional distance to your office. You can also walk more at work. Simply using the stairs rather than an elevator to move from floor to floor adds to your daily activity. Another consideration is whether your work facility is spread across several buildings. For example, I am employed at a large urban university that has a spacious campus. During each day I often have meetings in buildings on different parts of the campus, and I walk to these meetings. By the time I move from one building to another building and return, I usually walk a mile or more. Adding more walking is an easy way to add physical activity to your daily routine, but you may ask yourself whether these small walking periods each day yield health benefits. You bet they do! Some of these daily activity additions seem small, but when all are put together, they add up to major amounts of physical activity that moves you toward increased daily activity and important health benefits.

Another means to increase your daily physical activity is to engage in hobbies or activities that you enjoy such as walking the dog, doing yard work, gardening, or doing carpentry. Is walking the dog really good for you? The answer is yes, and walking is also good for the dog. What about mowing the lawn and working in the garden? Again, the answer is yes for both, although if you ride the lawn mower or you sit while doing the garden work you will do little physical activity and will not gain health benefits. In addition, physical activity must reach a certain intensity level to provide health benefits. As we discussed in chapter 3, the exercise intensity for reaching health benefits must be at least moderate, but vigorous physical activity can result in greater health benefits than moderate physical activity.

Let's consider for a minute the concept of activity intensity. The three levels of intensity are light, moderate, and vigorous.

- Light physical activity is any activity more strenuous than sleeping and less strenuous than a brisk walk.

- Moderate physical activity is represented by activities such as brisk walking and is about three to six *metabolic equivalents (METs)* of work. Metabolic equivalents are a measurement of work and the body's ability to consume oxygen. One MET is equal to the amount of oxygen consumed at rest. When doing moderate activity, you should be able to walk at a pace of three to four miles per hour.

- Vigorous physical activity is any activity that requires work greater than six METs. This kind of activity includes jogging at a pace greater than five miles per hour.

Regular involvement in moderate and vigorous physical activities provides important health benefits as discussed in chapter 3, and all of the activities discussed in this chapter are either moderate or vigorous in intensity and result in health gains. With this information in mind, let's set your first short-term goal. This goal should focus on changing your daily routines so that you increase your physical activity.

Your first short-term goal is to modify your lifestyle and incorporate more walking into your daily activities during the next two weeks.

This goal can be easily accomplished by parking your car farther away from your workplace and using the stairs rather than the elevator. Don't limit yourself to adding activity at your place of work, though. You can also increase your daily physical activity when going to places such as shopping malls. At a mall you can park your car at quite a distance from where you enter the mall, and when you move from floor to floor of the mall use the stairs.

Planning an Exercise Program

Even though you have set a goal to incorporate physical activity into your lifestyle, you should also devise a planned exercise program in order to increase your physical fitness and to meet your long-term goal of expending 1,500 kcal of energy each week. When developing an exercise program, you should consider the following fitness components: cardiovascular fitness, muscular fitness, flexibility, and body composition. After discussing the components, we'll talk about the parts of an exercise session and four exercise principles that are important in planning a program.

Cardiovascular fitness, also referred to as aerobic fitness or aerobic capacity, is developed by focusing on exercises that enhance the function of your heart, circulatory system, lungs, and skeletal muscles all at the same time. When cardiovascular fitness is high, so is aerobic capacity. For maximum effectiveness, cardiovascular conditioning should include exercises that are rhythmic, continuous, and involve the large muscle groups (primarily located in the lower part of your body). Walking, jogging, cycling, aerobic dance, and stair climbing are examples of exercises that use large muscle groups and can enhance your heart function, cardiovascular fitness, and aerobic capacity. Activities combining upper- and lower-body movements such as cross-country skiing, rowing, walking, jogging, running, and swimming can lead to even higher aerobic capacity.

Muscular fitness is enhanced by resistance training. Here the focus of the exercise is to enhance skeletal muscular strength and endurance. Exercises used in this type of training can emphasize strength, endurance, or both. When your goal is to increase strength and size of muscles, you should lift a weight 6 to 8 times, or repetitions (reps), before becoming fatigued to the point that you are unable to continue. On the other hand, if your goal is to increase muscular endurance, you should lift a weight 12 to 15 reps before fatiguing.

There are two facts to keep in mind. First, unless muscular strength and endurance exercises are performed regularly, you will lose up to half a pound of muscle for every year of life after age 25. Second, muscle is very active tissue with high energy requirements. Even when you are asleep, your muscles are responsible for more than 25 percent of your body's use of kilocalories. An increase in muscle tissue causes a corresponding increase in the number of kilocalories your body burns, even at rest.

Flexibility is the ability for muscles to move joints through their full range of motion, and it is a critical element that is often overlooked in exercise programs. Being able to use a joint's full range of motion can increase physical performance, decrease risk of injury, increase that particular joint's blood supply, improve balance, decrease risk of pain such as in the low back, and reduce muscular stress.

Body composition is also a component of physical fitness and refers to the two basic tissues found in the body: lean mass (muscle, bone, vital tissues, and organs) and fat mass. An optimal ratio of fat to lean mass is used by some as an indication of fitness, and with the right amount of appropriate exercises you can decrease body fat while increasing muscle mass.

Exercise Sessions

A planned exercise session has three basic components: the warm-up, the cardiovascular fitness and muscular fitness portion, and the cool-down. Each of these components can vary in length depending on what your goals are. Here we will discuss the warm-up and cool-down, and later in this chapter we'll take an in-depth look at the cardiovascular and muscular fitness portion.

The warm-up is the first part of the exercise session. It is important because it increases the body's temperature. A common mistake made by many people just starting an exercise program is overstretching or doing too many range-of-motion exercises before the muscles are adequately warmed up. Never stretch a cold muscle; rather, warm up the body by doing light aerobic exercises. The best time to stretch your muscles is after they are warm. One way of warming the body is by doing the same activity that you do during the cardiovascular fitness portion of the exercise session, but at a much lower intensity. This warm-up exercise can be an easy walk or an activity at less than 40 percent of your maximum heart rate (HRmax) (see page 66). The warm-up should last from 5 to 10 minutes. After finishing your warm-up exercises, your muscles should be warm, which may help prevent injury.

The cool-down portion of an exercise session is similar to the warm-up in that it should last 5 to 10 minutes and should be done at a low intensity (40 to 50 percent of HRmax). After you have completed the cardiovascular and muscular fitness portion of the session, the cool-down portion begins. This part of the exercise session is extremely important for developing flexibility because it is where you gain the most benefits from flexibility and range-of-motion exercises. With increased flexibility, your performance levels are likely to be higher and your injury risk reduced. Later in the chapter we'll describe and illustrate some effective flexibility exercises.

Range-of-motion and flexibility exercises are best performed moving through the full range of motion slowly. When you reach the farthest point in the movement, hold at that point for six to eight seconds. This form of stretching is referred to as static stretching and is different from ballistic stretching. Ballistic stretching uses the same stretching position, but movement is performed faster and is not held when the farthest movement point is reached. As a result, the movement looks as though bouncing is incorporated, which is why it is called ballistic stretching. This form of stretching can cause tears in the muscle tissue and other tissue damage and is not recommended.

It is a good idea to add two exercises to the cool-down: push-ups and abdominal curls. These are not flexibility exercises—instead they enhance strength and endurance—but they take little time and can be done without any added expense. Doing push-ups increases the tone of the muscles in the upper extremities, including the pectoral, deltoid, biceps, and triceps muscles. Abdominal curls will increase the tone of the muscles in the abdominal area, including the rectus abdominis and external obliques.

Exercise Principles

Whether your interest is in cardiovascular fitness or muscular fitness, four keys to selecting the right kinds of exercises for each of the basic components of fitness are found in the following principles.

• *Overload.* This principle implies that you must work at a level of moderate to vigorous exercise intensity long enough to overload your body above its resting level in order to bring about improvement.

• *Progression.* This principle means that when starting an exercise program, it is better to start at lower intensity, frequency, and duration and over several weeks or months slowly progress to higher exercise intensities of longer durations and at a greater frequency.

• *Specificity.* Exercise training is specific, and this principle means that you need to select the type of activities that will help you meet your long-term goal. For example, because one of your goals is to reduce blood cholesterol and because the best way to positively affect blood cholesterol is to choose activities that improve cardiovascular fitness, you need to select activities like walking, running, or biking. An exercise program that primarily focuses on muscular fitness is not the best program for moving toward your goal of achieving a healthy blood lipid and lipoprotein profile.

• *Reversibility.* You can't save up cardiovascular fitness. Once you have reached a desirable fitness level, at least two or three exercise sessions a week are necessary to maintain the achieved fitness level.

Cardiovascular Exercise Program

How often, how long, and how hard you exercise and what kinds of exercises you do should be determined by your goals and what you are trying to accomplish in developing an exercise program. Your goals, present fitness level, age, health, and interest along with consideration given to convenience are among the factors you should consider as you develop your personal exercise prescription. When your goal is to develop cardiovascular fitness and form a more favorable cholesterol and lipoprotein profile, four guiding principles can help you. For maximum effectiveness and safety in developing cardiovascular fitness, the exercise prescription should consider frequency, intensity, duration, and type of exercise (mode).

Frequency

When beginning the program, you should plan to exercise at least three days per week, and as your cardiovascular fitness improves, you can progress to four, five, or more days per week. This progression in the frequency of exercise is consistent with the surgeon general's exercise recommendations for improving cardiovascular fitness (DHHS 1996). In regards to improving and maintaining muscular fitness, you should complete resistance exercise training one to two times per week.

Intensity

Exercise intensity refers to the pace at which you walk, jog, pedal a bike, or swim. Two indicators of exercise intensity are your heart rate and your perception of the work rate. First, though, you need to determine your maximum heart rate.

Determining Maximum Heart Rate

Maximum heart rate (HRmax) is the highest rate at which your heart can contract. In developing an exercise prescription, use your maximum heart rate to determine exercise intensity. Generally, two ways exist for determining your maximum heart rate. The first method is more complicated and involves completing a maximal exercise test. A less complicated method is to predict your maximum heart rate using the following formula.

Let's use an example where the age of the person is 50:

$$\text{Predicted HRmax} = 220 - \text{age}$$
$$\text{HRmax} = 220 - 50$$
$$\text{HRmax} = 170$$

Measuring Your Heart Rate

Your training heart rate zone is a critical element in determining exercise intensity. Counting your pulse and determining your heart rate during an exercise session is one of the primary ways to ascertain the intensity at which you are working. There are many ways to measure exercise intensity, but, as mentioned, heart rate is widely accepted as a good method for measuring intensity during running, swimming, cycling, and other aerobic activities. The heart rate you should maintain is called your target heart rate. One of the simplest methods for determining this target is to calculate your predicted maximum heart rate as done in the previous section. Multiply the predicted maximum heart rate by the exercise intensity (as a decimal) at which you want to exercise.

Earlier in this chapter we defined moderate physical activity and vigorous physical activity. For improved aerobic fitness, ACSM recommends that exercise intensity be moderate to vigorous. If you are a beginner, you should start your program at a moderate intensity, such as 40 or 50 percent of HRmax, and over a period of weeks or months work toward vigorous exercise intensities of 60 to 70 percent of HRmax. If you start your planned exercise program at a moderate intensity of 40 percent, over time you can progress up to vigorous exercise intensities of 70 or even 80 percent (ACSM 2005).

Here's an example of determining target heart rate, using 50 as the age and 70 percent, or vigorous activity, as the intensity:

$$\text{Target exercise heart rate} = (220 - \text{age}) \times 70 \text{ percent}$$
$$\text{Target exercise heart rate} = (220 - 50) \times 0.70$$
$$\text{Target exercise heart rate} = (170) \times 0.70$$
$$\text{Target exercise heart rate} = 119$$

Other methods exist for calculating your target rate that consider individual resting heart rate differences. These calculations have been completed and are included in table 5.1.

Table 5.1   Target Heart Rates for Different Ages

Intensity (percent)	Age			
	40	50	60	70
50	90	85	80	75
60	108	102	96	90
70	126	119	112	105
80	144	136	128	120

In order to determine your resting heart rate you will need a digital watch or a watch with a second hand. After sitting quietly for five minutes, count your heart rate for 10 seconds and multiply by six to get the per-minute rate. You count heart rate by palpating your pulse on the radial artery. With the palm of your left hand facing up, place the index and middle finger of your right hand over the artery that is near the surface next to the tendons on your left wrist (see figure 5.1). Do the same procedure immediately after exercise, and you will have your exercise heart rate.

Another procedure for counting heart rate requires the purchase of a heart rate monitor that straps around your chest and is more accurate. The monitor will give you feedback on a digital watch that tells you exactly what your heart rate is at any time during the exercise session or when at rest.

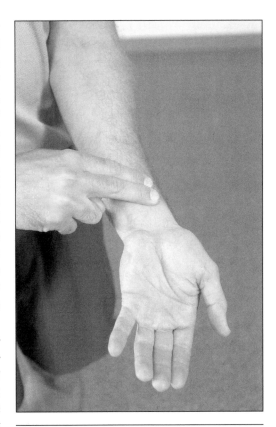

Figure 5.1 Determining heart rate by taking a pulse at the wrist.

Measuring Perception of Work Rate

The scale for the Borg Rating of Perceived Exertion (RPE) was developed to help people get in touch with their level of exertion and how they feel when exercising. Higher exercise levels that result in higher levels of energy expenditure and physiological stress result in higher RPE ratings. For example, when at rest you would rate your exertion as very, very light, or a 6 or 7 on the scale in figure 5.2. This number has also been related to heart rate. An RPE rating of 13 or 14 corresponds with a heart rate of 130 or 140 and is perceived as somewhat hard. You should learn to judge how your body feels when you exercise and set a goal for an RPE of 13 or 14—somewhat hard—which means you are exercising at a moderate intensity. In this sense you're learning to listen to how your body is responding to exercise.

6	No exertion at all
7	
8	Extremely light
9	Very light
10	
11	Light
12	
13	Somewhat hard
14	
15	Hard (heavy)
16	
17	Very hard
18	
19	Extremely hard
20	Maximal exertion

Borg RPE scale
© Gunnar Borg, 1970, 1985, 1994, 1998

Figure 5.2 Borg's Rating of Perceived Exertion scale.

G. Borg, 1998, *Borg's perceived exertion and pain scales* (Champaign, IL: Human Kinetics), 47.

Duration

Exercise duration refers to the amount of time the exercise session lasts. Initially, exercise duration should be 15 to 20 minutes. Over several months, duration can progress to 30, 40, or more minutes per session. This time period does not include the warm-up and cool-down portions of the exercise session, which should last about 10 to 20 minutes each. Another consideration in developing your exercise program is whether you want to split the aerobic exercise into multiple sessions. For instance, you can have two 15-minute exercise sessions at different points in the day for a total of 30 minutes of aerobic exercise. As previously mentioned, spreading 30 minutes of exercise throughout the day has been proven to be as effective as one 30-minute session (Donnelly et al. 2000). Note that to get the most positive changes in your blood lipid profile, you need to work toward longer times spent doing endurance exercise.

Type

Type refers to the mode of exercise you choose. In developing cardiovascular or aerobic fitness, you have many different modes of exercise to select from, such as walking, swimming, or bicycling. Perhaps you have heard people say that there is one best type of exercise for everyone. It's true, there is a best exercise for everyone—the exercise that you enjoy and will continue throughout your life. Keep in mind, though, that whatever mode you choose, you still want to measure how much energy you are burning during your activity. Use the sidebar on page 69 to help you determine this expenditure.

Kilocalories: Measuring Energy Expenditure

Kilocalories are units of energy. One kcal, also referred to as one large calorie or 1,000 calories, is used to define the energy value of foods and energy expenditure. Kilocalories are often used as a means for understanding how much we eat, but we can also use kilocalories to better understand how much we exercise. For example, a person exercising at eight minutes per mile and weighing 150 pounds can expend energy worth 426 kcals in 30 minutes. For other selected exercises and the kilocalories used, see table 5.2. The information in this table is categorized by type of exercise, time spent exercising, and body weight.

Table 5.2 Energy Expenditure in Kilocalories for Selected Activities

Weight (pounds)	Length of exercise session (minutes)	Walking 2.0 mph	Walking 3.0 mph	Walking 4.0 mph	Jogging 12 min per mile	Jogging 10 min per mile	Jogging 8 min per mile	Swimming Slow crawl	Cycling 5.5 mph	Cycling 9.4 mph
105	15	36	54	69	87	126	147	90	45	72
	30	72	108	138	174	252	294	180	90	144
	45	108	162	207	261	378	441	270	135	216
125	15	45	63	81	105	146	179	108	54	84
	30	90	126	162	210	291	357	216	108	168
	45	135	189	243	315	437	536	324	162	252
150	15	54	75	99	126	180	213	131	66	102
	30	108	150	198	252	360	426	261	132	204
	45	162	225	297	378	540	639	392	198	306
175	15	63	89	117	150	214.5	247.5	153	77	120
	30	126	177	234	300	429	495	306	153	240
	45	189	266	351	450	644	743	459	230	360
200	15	72	102	132	171	250.5	283.5	177	88.5	138
	30	144	204	264	342	501	567	354	177	276
	45	216	306	396	513	751.5	850.5	531	265.5	414
225	15	81	112.5	145.5	192	267	309	193.5	97.5	150
	30	162	225	291	384	534	618	387	195	300
	45	243	337.5	436.5	576	801	927	580.5	292.5	450

The energy expenditure data are copyright © Fitness Technologies Inc., and may not be reproduced or copied in any form without permission of Fitness Technologies Press. 5043 Via Lara Lane. Santa Barbara, CA 93111. Adapted from McArdle WD, Katch FI, Katch VL. *Exercise Physiology: Energy, Nutrition, and Human Performance.* 5th edition. Williams & Wilkins. Baltimore, 2001.

Setting Short-Term Cardiovascular Fitness Goals

To achieve optimal cardiovascular fitness, the ACSM recommends an exercise frequency of three to five or more times per week (ACSM 2005). As a general rule for beginners, you should space your exercise sessions throughout the week on nonconsecutive days, which provides time for you to recover between sessions. As time passes and you gain cardiovascular fitness, you can exercise on consecutive days, but even after you have been exercising for several months, avoid consecutive days of hard exercise. Your body needs time to recover, and when you are exercising five or more days a week, you should have easy days in between hard days.

The ACSM also recommends that the exercise intensity be moderate to vigorous. Again, beginners should start a program at a moderate exercise intensity, say 40 or 50 percent of HRmax, and over a period of weeks to months slowly increase how hard they work toward vigorous exercise intensities of 60 to 70 percent HRmax. The duration should be approximately 20 to 60 minutes. Beginners should set an exercise duration goal of 20 minutes, and after several months, that goal should be increased to 30 minutes and then 40 minutes or more (see table 5.3 for a comprehensive exercise program for beginners). For optimal exercise programming that will positively change your blood lipid and lipoprotein profile, the greater the exercise volume the better. After you have been working on your planned exercise program for several months, your exercise duration goal should include sessions that last 45 minutes or more each (see table 5.4 for an exercise program for individuals who have already been exercising).

> Your first short-term goal in developing an exercise program is to engage in three planned cardiovascular sessions per week for the next three weeks and then increase to four sessions per week.

Muscular Fitness Exercise Program

As we start to discuss goals and the prescription of exercise for muscular fitness, remember that enhancing muscular fitness does have many health benefits, but the overall effect on the cholesterol and lipoprotein profile is not as great as that associated with cardiovascular fitness. Having said this, all of the previously discussed exercise principles for cardiovascular fitness also apply to developing muscular fitness. Earlier in this chapter, two different types of muscular fitness were defined: strength and endurance. When your muscular fitness goal is endurance development, your exercise training should emphasize a higher number of repetitions (8 to 12 or even 15 reps) completed with each set. On the other hand, if strength

Table 5.3 **Sample Exercise Program for Beginners**

Week	Sunday	Monday	Tuesday	Wednesday	Thursday	Friday	Saturday
1	1-mile walk,* stretch	Resistance training (lower body): 5 exercises, 1 set per exercise, 8-12 RM**	1-mile walk, stretch	Rest	Resistance training (upper body): 5 exercises, 1 set per exercise, 8-12 RM	Rest	1-mile walk, stretch
2	Rest	1-mile walk, stretch	Rest	Resistance training (lower body): 5 exercises, 1 set per exercise, 8-12 RM	1-mile walk, stretch	1-mile walk, stretch	Resistance training (upper body): 5 exercises, 1 set per exercise, 8-12 RM
3	1-mile walk, stretch	Rest	Resistance training (lower body): 5 exercises, 1 set per exercise, 8-12 RM	1-mile walk, stretch	Rest	Resistance training (upper body): 5 exercises, 1 set per exercise, 8-12 RM	1-mile walk, stretch
4	Rest	2-mile walk, stretch	Rest	Resistance training (lower body): 5 exercises, 1 set per exercise, 8-12 RM	2-mile walk, stretch	Resistance training (upper body): 5 exercises, 1 set per exercise, 8-12 RM	1-mile walk, stretch
5	2-mile walk, stretch	Rest	Any other activity***	Resistance training (lower body): 5 exercises, 1 set per exercise, 8-12 RM	Rest	3-mile walk, stretch	Resistance training (upper body): 5 exercises, 1 set per exercise, 8-12 RM

(continued)

Table 5.3 (continued)

Week	Sunday	Monday	Tuesday	Wednesday	Thursday	Friday	Saturday
6	Rest	2-mile walk, stretch	3-mile walk, stretch	Resistance training (lower body): 5 exercises, 1 set per exercise, 8-12 RM	Rest	2-mile walk, stretch	Resistance training (upper body): 5 exercises, 1 set per exercise, 8-12 RM
7	3-mile walk, stretch	2-mile walk, stretch	Rest	Resistance training (upper body): 5 exercises, 1 set per exercise, 8-12 RM	1-mile walk, stretch	Resistance training (lower body): 5 exercises, 1 set per exercise, 8-12 RM	Rest
8	Any other activity	2-mile walk, stretch	Resistance training (upper body): 5 exercises, 1 set per exercise, 8-12 RM	Rest	Resistance training (lower body): 5 exercises, 1 set per exercise, 8-12 RM	1-mile walk, stretch	Rest
9	3-mile walk, stretch	2-mile walk, stretch	Resistance training (upper body): 5 exercises, 1 set per exercise, 8-12 RM	Any other activity	Rest	Resistance training (lower body): 5 exercises, 1 set per exercise, 8-12 RM	Rest
10	Any other activity	2-mile walk, stretch	Rest	3-mile walk, stretch	Resistance training (upper body): 5 exercises, 1 set per exercise, 8-12 RM	Rest	Resistance training (lower body): 5 exercises, 1 set per exercise, 8-12 RM

Table 5.3 (continued)

Week	Sunday	Monday	Tuesday	Wednesday	Thursday	Friday	Saturday
11	3-mile walk, stretch	Resistance training (upper body): 5 exercises, 1 set per exercise, 8-12 RM	2-mile walk, stretch	Rest	Resistance training (lower body): 5 exercises, 1 set per exercise, 8-12 RM	Rest	Any other activity
12	3-mile walk, stretch	Rest	Resistance training (upper body): 5 exercises, 1 set per exercise, 8-12 RM	Any other activity	Rest	4-mile walk, stretch	Resistance training (lower body): 5 exercises, 1 set per exercise, 8-12 RM

Includes information from Feigenbaum, Matthew S. Exercise Prescription for Healthy Adults. In *Resistance Training for Health and Rehabilitation*, p. 107, edited by James E. Graves and Barry A. Franklin. Human Kinetics, 2001.

*Appropriate speeds are walking at 2 to 4 mph or jogging at a 12-minute-mile pace.

**8 to 12 RM (repetition maximum) = the maximum amount of weight that can be lifted for 8 to 12 reps.

***Other activities include cycling or swimming.

Upper-Body Exercises

1. Abdominal crunches or rotation crunches
2. Biceps curls or preacher curls
3. Triceps extensions or triceps presses
4. Chest presses or butterflies
5. Lat pull-downs, upright rows, pull-ups, or shoulder shrugs

Lower-Body Exercises

1. Seated leg curls or lying leg curls
2. Leg extensions
3. Leg presses or hack squats
4. Lunges or step-ups
5. Back extensions (on platform or machine)

Note: These exercises are meant to provide a comprehensive exercise prescription. This prescription is based on ACSM guidelines for exercise prescription to provide maximum benefits for muscular fitness.

The goal of this training plan is not to emphasize improvement in muscle mass; rather the goal is to provide a comprehensive exercise program that will enhance muscle strength and endurance. In order to accomplish this goal, the recommendation is to use a lower number of sets coupled with a higher number of reps per set with low weight.

Table 5.4 Sample Exercise Program for Intermediate Exercisers

Week	Sunday	Monday	Tuesday	Wednesday	Thursday	Friday	Saturday
1	5-mile walk,* stretch	Rest	Resistance training (upper body): 5 exercises, 1 set per exercise, 8-12 RM** 1-mile walk	Any other activity***	Rest	5-mile walk, stretch	Resistance training (lower body): 5 exercises, 1 set per exercise, 8-12 RM 1-mile walk
2	3-mile walk, stretch	Resistance training (upper body): 5 exercises, 1 set per exercise, 8-12 RM 1-mile walk	3-mile walk, stretch	Rest	Resistance training (lower body): 5 exercises, 1 set per exercise, 8-12 RM 1-mile walk	Rest	3-mile walk, stretch
3	Rest	3-mile walk, stretch	Rest	Resistance training (upper body): 5 exercises, 1 set per exercise, 8-12 RM 1-mile walk	3-mile walk, stretch	3-mile walk, stretch	Resistance training (lower body): 5 exercises, 1 set per exercise, 8-12 RM 1-mile walk
4	3-mile walk, stretch	Rest	Resistance training (upper body): 5 exercises, 1 set per exercise, 8-12 RM 1-mile walk	3-mile walk, stretch	Rest	Resistance training (lower body): 5 exercises, 1 set per exercise, 8-12 RM 1-mile walk	3-mile walk, stretch
5	Rest	5-mile walk, stretch	Rest	Resistance training (upper body): 5 exercises, 1 set per exercise, 8-12 RM 1-mile walk	4-mile walk	Resistance training (lower body): 5 exercises, 1 set per exercise, 8-12 RM 1-mile walk	3-mile walk, stretch

Table 5.4 (continued)

Week	Sunday	Monday	Tuesday	Wednesday	Thursday	Friday	Saturday
6	5-mile walk, stretch	Rest	Any other activity	Resistance training (upper body): 5 exercises, 1 set per exercise, 8-12 RM 1-mile walk	Rest	5-mile walk, stretch	Resistance training (lower body): 5 exercises, 1 set per exercise, 8-12 RM 1-mile walk
7	Rest	4-mile walk, stretch	5-mile walk, stretch	Resistance training (lower body): 5 exercises, 1 set per exercise, 8-12 RM 1-mile walk	Rest	5-mile walk, stretch	Resistance training (upper body): 5 exercises, 1 set per exercise, 8-12 RM 1-mile walk
8	5-mile walk, stretch	5-mile walk, stretch	Rest	Resistance training (lower body): 5 exercises, 1 set per exercise, 8-12 RM 1-mile walk	3-mile walk, stretch	Resistance training (upper body): 5 exercises, 1 set per exercise, 8-12 RM 1-mile walk	Rest
9	Any other activity	5-mile walk, stretch	Resistance training (lower body): 5 exercises, 1 set per exercise, 8-12 RM 1-mile walk	Rest	Resistance training (upper body): 5 exercises, 1 set per exercise, 8-12 RM 1-mile walk	3-mile walk, stretch	Rest
10	5-mile walk, stretch	5-mile walk, stretch	Resistance training (lower body): 5 exercises, 1 set per exercise, 8-12 RM 1-mile walk	Any other activity	Rest	Resistance training (upper body): 5 exercises, 1 set per exercise, 8-12 RM 1-mile walk	Rest

(continued)

Table 5.4 (continued)

Week	Sunday	Monday	Tuesday	Wednesday	Thursday	Friday	Saturday
11	Any other activity	5-mile walk, stretch	Rest	4-mile walk, stretch	Resistance training (lower body): 5 exercises, 1 set per exercise, 8-12 RM 1-mile walk	Rest	Resistance training (upper body): 5 exercises, 1 set per exercise, 8-12 RM 1-mile walk
12	5-mile walk, stretch	Resistance training (lower body): 5 exercises, 1 set per exercise, 8-12 RM 1-mile walk	5-mile walk, stretch	Rest	Resistance training (upper body): 5 exercises, 1 set per exercise, 8-12 RM 15 min of aerobic exercise	Rest	Any other activity

Includes information from Feigenbaum, Matthew S. Exercise Prescription for Healthy Adults. In *Resistance Training for Health and Rehabilitation*, p. 107, edited by James E. Graves and Barry A. Franklin. Human Kinetics, 2001.

*Appropriate speeds are walking at 2 to 4 mph or jogging at a 12-minute-mile pace.
**8 to 12 RM (repetition maximum) = the maximum amount of weight that can be lifted for 8 to 12 reps.
***Other activities include cycling and swimming.

Upper-Body Exercises

1. Abdominal crunches or rotation crunches
2. Biceps curls or preacher curls
3. Triceps extensions or triceps presses
4. Chest presses or butterflies
5. Lat pull-downs, upright rows, pull-ups, or shoulder shrugs

Lower-Body Exercises

1. Seated leg curls or lying leg curls
2. Leg extensions
3. Leg presses or hack squats
4. Lunges or step-ups
5. Back extensions (on platform or machine)

Note: These exercises are meant to provide a comprehensive exercise prescription for healthy adults. This prescription is based on ACSM guidelines for exercise prescription to provide maximum benefits for muscular fitness.

The goal of this training plan is not to emphasize improvement in muscle mass; rather the goal is to provide a comprehensive exercise program that will enhance strength and muscle endurance. In order to accomplish this goal, the recommendation is to use a lower number of sets coupled with a higher number of reps per set with low weight.

development is your goal, then a lower number of repetitions (6 to 8 reps) should be completed with each set. In order to optimize your blood cholesterol and lipoprotein profile, your goal should be the development of muscular fitness.

An endless array of strength training programs and theories is available, much of it geared toward bodybuilders and advanced exercisers. If you're just getting started, it's quite easy to become confused by all of the anatomical terms and gym jargon. We'll fill in the gap by giving you the foundation of a safe and effective strength training routine. You will learn about the major muscle groups and the exercises that target them, the difference between sets and reps, proper form, and the basics of frequency and progression.

Circuits, Sets, and Repetitions

A circuit is a group of exercises (usually five to eight) that work different muscle groups. Completing a circuit means doing an exercise for each major muscle group in the body. A set is a group of successive repetitions performed without a rest period. Repetitions, or reps, are the number of times you repeat a lift in each set. If you were to do three sets of 12 biceps curls, you would curl the weight 12 times in a row to complete the first set. Then you'd put the weight down, rest a moment or two, and do 12 more reps to complete the second set. Finally, you'd do the set a third time so that you finished the three prescribed exercise sets. If you're working out with a friend, your rest interval between sets is the amount of time it takes for your partner to finish a set. This rest interval is rarely more than about a minute and a half. If you are not exercising with anyone, the rest period is usually about 45 seconds to a minute in length. Other exercise professionals may recommend longer rest periods. These recommendations are fine because the longer rest period is most likely based on a program that will result in greater strength gains.

Proper Form

Proper form includes speed and movement through a full range of motion. Speed of movement is an important element of each exercise. A reasonable training pace is two to four seconds each for the lifting (*concentric*) portion and for the lowering (*eccentric*) portion of the exercise. Fast, jerky movements should be avoided; such movements place undue stress on muscle and connective tissue and substantially increase the likelihood for injury. Fast lifting also cheats you out of some strength benefits by developing momentum. As a result, the momentum, not the muscle, does much of the work, and your muscles gain little benefit.

Another important aspect of proper form is movement through a full range of motion. Each exercise movement should be taken through the complete range of the joint's movement in a controlled manner. If a weight is so heavy that you have to jerk, bounce, or swing to get it to the top of the movement, you are lifting too much weight. These types of movements compromise form and reduce gains in optimal muscular strength and endurance.

Frequency, Duration, and Intensity

To attain muscular endurance benefits, the ACSM recommends weight training two days per week (frequency), performing one to three sets of 8 to 12 reps (duration) of eight to ten different exercises at approximately 70 to 85 percent of your *one-repetition maximum,* or 1RM (intensity) (ACSM 2005). 1RM is the maximum amount of weight that you can lift one time (see the sidebar on this page for directions on determining your 1RM). You can use your 1RM to determine the amount of weight to lift for any exercise during normal resistance training. Following is an example of how to do this calculation. If the most weight that you can lift at one time is 50 pounds for a biceps curl and you want to train at 70 percent of that 1RM, you would change 70 percent to 0.70 and multiply that by your 1RM of 50 pounds to give you an exercise training weight of 35 pounds:

$$0.70 \times 50 \text{ pounds} = 35 \text{ pounds}$$

Using this equation allows you to estimate the amount of weight that you can lift for 6 to 12 reps. If you are unable to lift the weight at least six times, reduce the weight until you are able to lift it six or more times. On the other hand, if you are able to lift the weight more than 12 times, add a small amount of weight.

If you're just beginning an exercise program, start in the low range of the previous recommendations. For example, participate in a cardiovascular activity (e.g., walking, aerobics, cycling) for 20 minutes three times a week, and add strength training to your workout on two other days of the week. Schedule 48 hours of rest between your strength workouts to allow your muscles to recover after each exercise session.

Determining 1RM

To figure out your 1RM, or the highest amount of weight you can lift at one time, use the following procedure. Choose any typical exercise using free weights or a weight machine (for example, a biceps curl or a leg press). Perform one repetition of the exercise using a weight that you can lift easily. Rest for two or three minutes and then increase the weight by 5 to 10 pounds. Lift this new weight, rest, and repeat this process until you reach the highest weight you can lift while still maintaining proper form (ACSM 2005).

Target Exercises for Major Muscle Groups

When selecting exercises for your muscular fitness routine, it's important to include at least one exercise for each major muscle group. This prevents muscle imbalances that often lead to injury. Let's look at the major muscle groups and a few of the exercises that you can select to improve strength and endurance. These exercise descriptions and illustrations are provided later in the chapter.

- *Gluteals.* This group of muscles includes the gluteus maximus, which is the main muscle of the buttocks. Common exercises are squats and leg presses.
- *Quadriceps.* This group of muscles is found in the front part of the thigh. Exercises include squats, lunges, leg extensions, and leg presses.
- *Hamstrings.* These muscles make up the back of the thigh. Exercises include squats, lunges, leg presses, and leg curls.
- *Hip abductors and adductors.* These are the muscles of the inner and outer thigh. They can be worked with a variety of side-lying leg lifts, standing cable pulls, and machines that have multihip movements.
- *Calves.* The calf or gastrocnemius and soleus muscles are found on the back of the lower leg. Standing calf raises and seated or bent-knee calf raises will work this muscle group.
- *Low back.* The erector spinae muscles extend the back and aid in good posture. Exercises include back-extension and prone back-extension exercises.
- *Abdominals.* These muscles include the rectus abdominis and external obliques. Exercises such as abdominal standard or rotation crunches and abdominal curls work this muscle group.
- *Pectoralis major.* This large, fan-shaped muscle is found in the front of the upper chest. Exercises include push-ups, pull-ups, and bench presses.
- *Rhomboids.* These muscles are in the middle of the upper back between the shoulder blades. They are worked in chin-ups, dumbbell bent rows, and other moves that bring the shoulder blades together.
- *Trapezius.* These muscles are found in the upper portion of the back, running from the neck to the shoulder. Exercises include upright rows and shoulder shrugs with resistance.
- *Latissimus dorsi.* These are the large muscles found in the midback. Exercises working these muscles include pull-ups, chin-ups, one-arm bent rows, dips on parallel bars, and lat pulldowns.

- *Deltoids.* These muscles are found on the top of the shoulder. Front, standing lateral, and rear dumbbell raises all target the deltoid.
- *Biceps.* These muscles are found in the front of the upper arm. The best exercises are biceps curls, which can be done with a barbell, dumbbells, or machines.
- *Triceps.* These muscles are found in the back of the upper arm. Exercises for this area include pushing movements like push-ups, dips, and triceps extensions.

Progression

Proper progression in resistance programs is achieved by adding weight, and it is the key to any well-designed muscular fitness program. This means that as your muscles adapt to a given exercise and weight, you need to gradually increase the resistance (the amount of weight lifted) or the number of reps in order to promote further fitness gains. You should start out with a weight that allows you to do at least 8 reps of a particular exercise. Once you can complete 12 reps or even 15 reps with that weight, you should increase the weight by about 5 percent but no more than 10 percent. Now, go back to doing 8 reps with the heavier weight. Once you've worked up to 12 reps with the heavier weight, you again increase the amount of weight by another 5 percent and return to doing 8 reps. Keep increasing reps and resistance and you will continue to see muscular fitness gains.

Increases in size and strength of muscles don't occur during the exercise session; they occur during the rest period between workouts. Recovery periods are when your muscles regenerate and rebuild, gradually becoming bigger and stronger. The recovery process can take at least 48 hours. For this reason, strength training should be scheduled no more frequently than every other day. If you prefer to train more often, avoid using the same muscle group on consecutive days. For example, you could do exercises for your upper body on one day and then exercises for your lower body the next day.

Setting Short-Term Muscular Fitness Goals

In this chapter we have already set one long-term goal, one short-term goal regarding daily physical activity, and one short-term goal regarding cardiovascular fitness. Now you need to consider developing a short-term goal for enhancing muscular fitness, but before starting work on this goal, consider waiting three to four weeks. The reason for delaying implementation of a muscular fitness program is that you have already increased your daily activity by starting a cardiovascular fitness program. Starting too many short-term goals at one time is not a characteristic for successful lifestyle behavior change. Thus, implementation of a muscular fitness program should be delayed until you have made significant gains toward your first two short-term goals of increasing daily activity and cardiovascular fitness.

Your first short-term goal for developing muscular fitness is to engage in two planned resistance exercise sessions per week for the next four weeks.

Resistance Training and Flexibility Exercises

Tables 5.3 and 5.4 on pages 71-76 contain sample programs for both cardiovascular and muscular fitness. You'll see that we've recommended a certain number of resistance exercises per session, according to muscle group. Following are instructions and photographs detailing the procedures for the exercises previously recommended for each muscle group. We also include descriptions and photos for 15 flexibility exercises, categorized by upper- and lower-body stretches. Use the photos to guide you in developing proper form.

QUADRICEPS STRETCH

With one hand on a nearby wall for support, grab one ankle and pull it up to the rear.

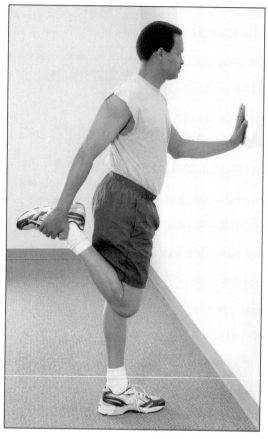

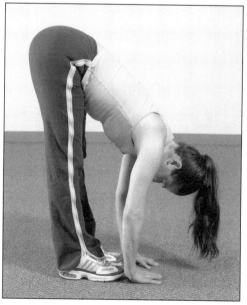

HAMSTRING STRETCH

With feet together, bend down and touch the toes or as close as possible.

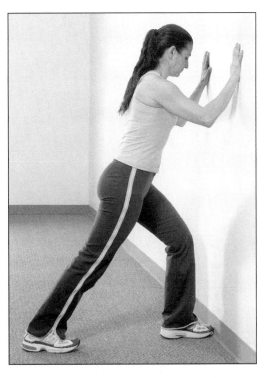

CALF STRETCH (WALL)

Place both hands on a wall, shoulder-width apart. Place one leg behind the other, being sure to keep the heel on the ground during the stretch. Bend the front knee, shifting the body weight forward.

CALF STRETCH (STAIRS)

Stand on a step. Using a handrail for support, keep one foot completely on the stair. Make sure the arch of the back foot rests on the stair. Shift weight onto the back foot.

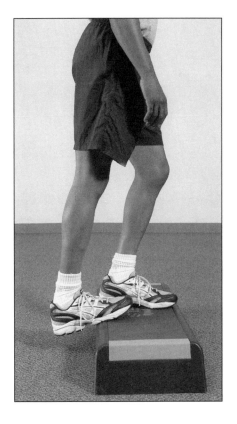

GASTROCNEMIUS STRETCH

Place one foot behind the other, keeping the heel on the floor. Place the hands on the front leg for support. Shift the body weight onto the front leg in a lunge-type fashion.

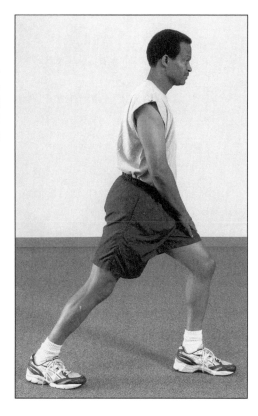

GROIN STRETCH

Sit on the floor and place the feet together in front of you. Allow the knees to lower to induce a stretch. Press down on the knees as needed for more stretch.

HURDLER STRETCH

While sitting on the floor, extend one leg in front of you. Tuck the opposite foot in toward the extended leg so the foot is near the knee. Reach forward with both hands and hold for several seconds, then relax. Be sure to keep your back straight.

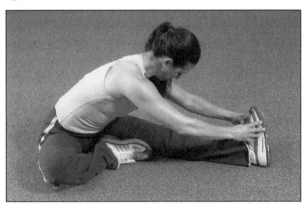

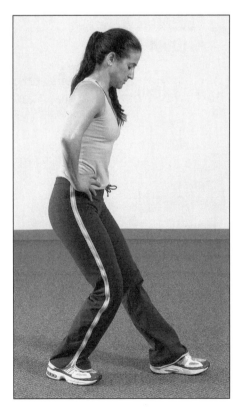

SOLEUS (ACHILLES TENDON) STRETCH

Stand with one foot behind the other. Keep the heel of the rear foot on the ground, distribute weight evenly over both feet, and bend the back knee. Place your hands on your hips for balance.

PECTORAL STRETCH

Place your hands on the back of the head, bring the elbows back, and hold.

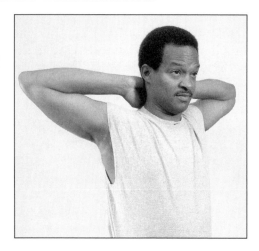

PECTORAL STRETCH (DOOR FRAME)

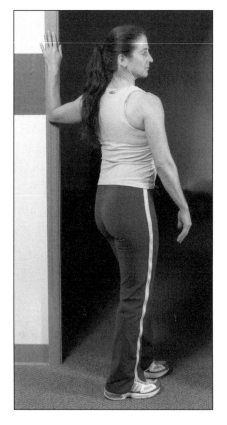

Place one hand on a door frame, turn the body away from the frame, and hold.

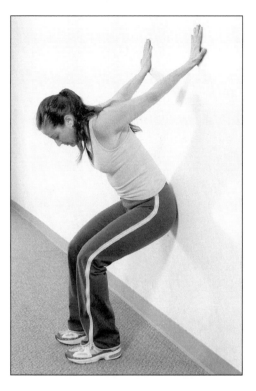

DELTOID STRETCH (WALL)

Facing away from a wall and bending over, place hands on the wall as high as possible with the fingers upward. Squat down until a stretch is felt and hold this position.

DELTOID STRETCH

Grab one elbow with the opposite hand and pull it across the chest until a stretch is felt. Hold this position.

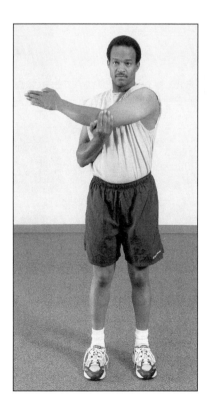

TRICEPS STRETCH

Hold one arm above the head, grab the elbow with the opposite hand, and pull it toward the head.

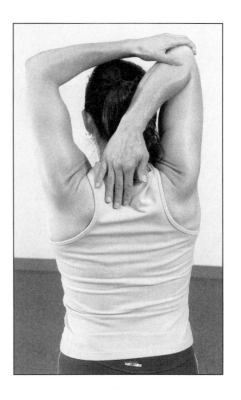

FOREARM STRETCH

Hold one arm straight out in front of you. Grab that hand with the other and pull it toward the shoulder until a stretch is felt.

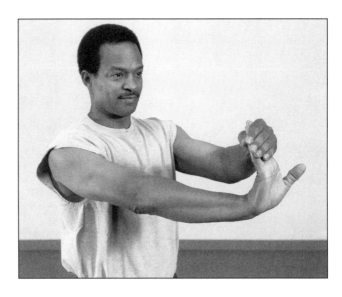

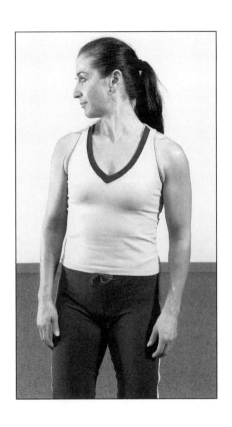

NECK STRETCH

Turn your head over one shoulder until a stretch is felt and hold that position. Repeat, turning your head to the other side.

PUSH-UP

Lying facedown on the floor with your arms shoulder-width apart and back completely straight, raise your body off the floor and fully extend your arms. Then slowly lower to the floor.

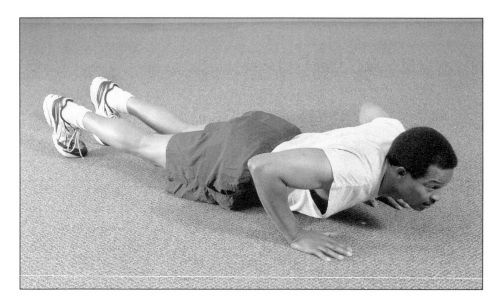

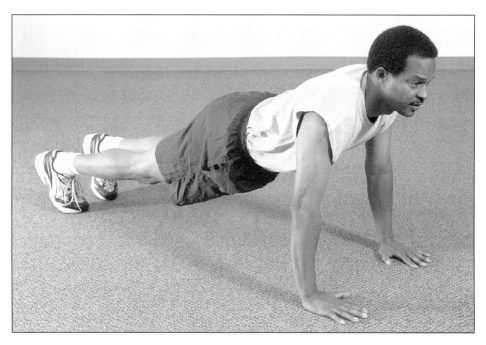

KNEE PUSH-UP

In the same position as a regular push-up, except with knees on the floor and legs crossed, keep your elbows near the body and your back straight. Raise your body slowly until your arms are fully extended, and slowly return to the starting position.

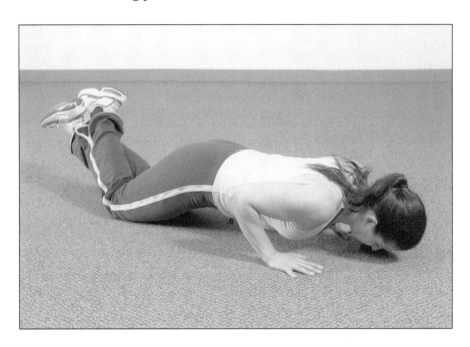

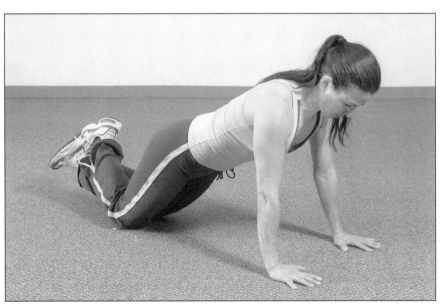

ABDOMINAL CURL

Lie on your back with your knees bent. With arms folded across the chest, raise the upper back and shoulders from the floor. Keep the lower back on the ground. Relax and slowly return to the starting position.

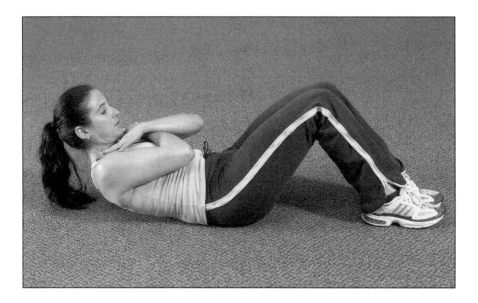

LEG PRESS (MACHINE)

Works the quadriceps

Place your feet on the platform shoulder-width apart and press up. Lower the safety catch and then lower the weight until the knees are at roughly a 60-degree angle. Then extend the legs until just before the knees lock.

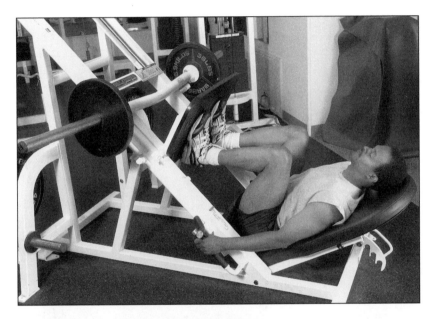

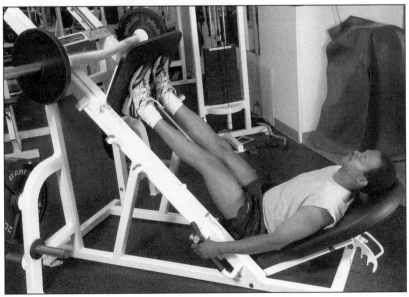

LUNGE WITH HAND WEIGHTS

Works the quadriceps

Hold a dumbbell in each hand. Step forward with one leg and make sure the heel of the leading foot hits first, then the toe. Lower the body until each leg has a 90-degree bend. Return to the starting position by retracting the lead leg and placing your feet shoulder-width apart.

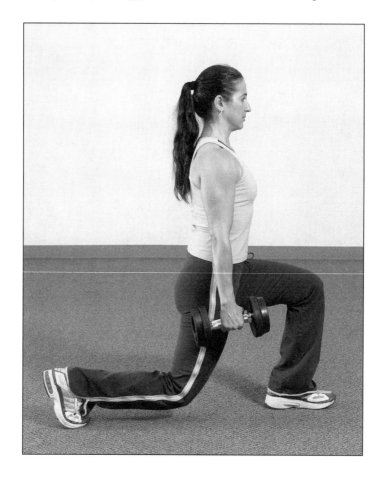

LEG EXTENSION (MACHINE)

Works the quadriceps

Place your legs behind the pad and extend them until they are straight. Slowly let the bar come back to its starting position.

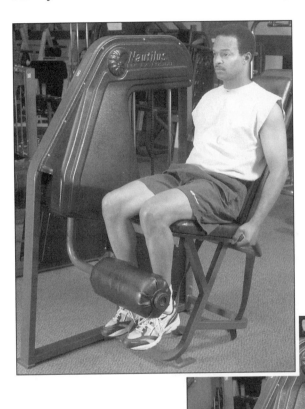

BARBELL SQUAT

Works the quadriceps

Hold a barbell with hands shoulder-width apart. Keeping the back straight, squat down so the knees are at about a 90-degree angle. Take care not to allow the knees to go past the toes.

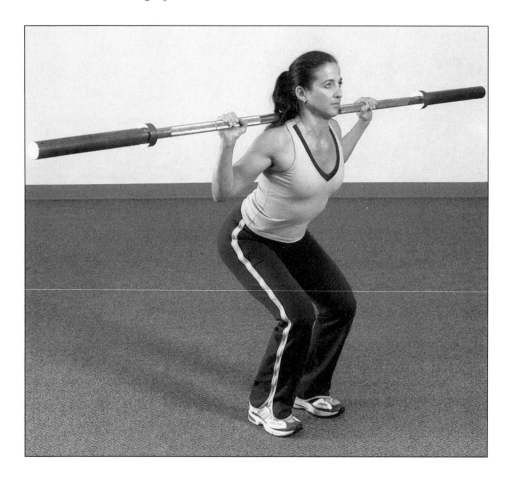

STEP-UP WITH HAND WEIGHTS

Works the quadriceps

Stand in front of an elevated platform. Step onto the platform in a slow, deliberate motion. Then step down in the same fashion.

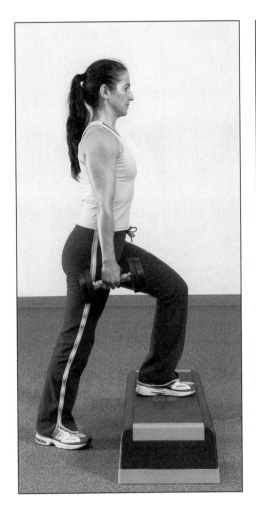
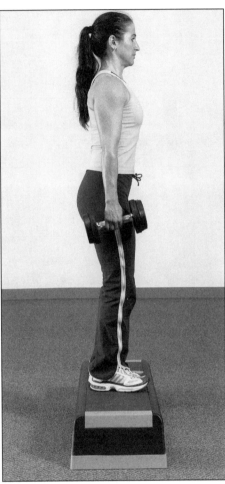

LYING LEG CURLS (MACHINE)

Works the hamstrings

Place your legs under the pad and pull up until the calves are vertical (past 90 degrees), then let the pad slowly return to starting position.

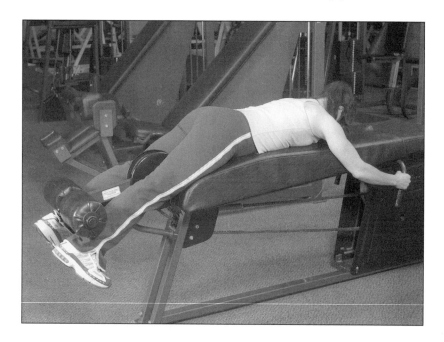

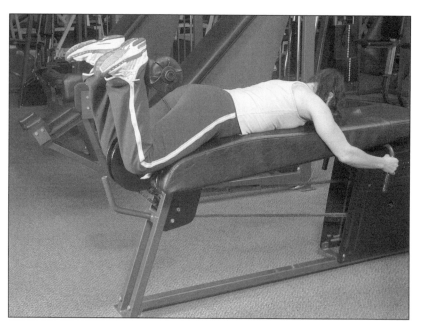

SEATED LEG CURLS (MACHINE)

Works the hamstrings

Place your legs on the pad and pull down until the pad almost reaches the thighs. Let the weight return slowly to starting position.

BACK EXTENSION ON PLATFORM

Works the erector spinae

Start with the body diagonal to the floor and with the back straight. Lower the upper body at the hips until a 90-degree angle is formed by the legs and back. Slowly raise the upper body back to a straight position.

BACK EXTENSION (MACHINE)

Works the erector spinae

Place your back against the pad while sitting. Press back until the back is hyperextended, then return slowly to the starting position.

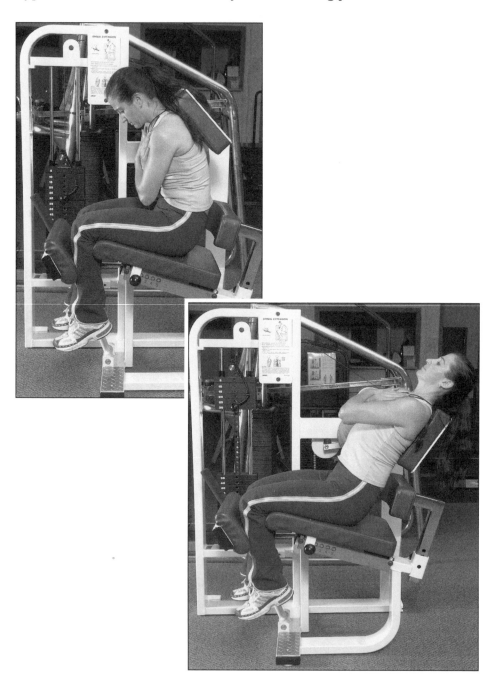

ABDOMINAL CRUNCHES

Works the rectus abdominis

Start by lying on your back with knees bent at a 90-degree angle. With the arms folded across the chest, lift the upper body and then lower it. This exercise can also be done on a machine.

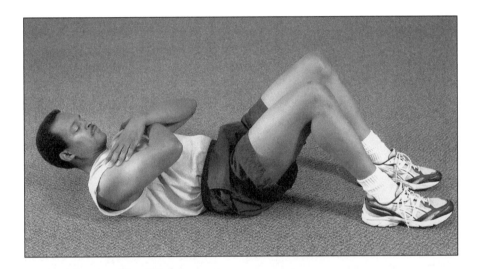

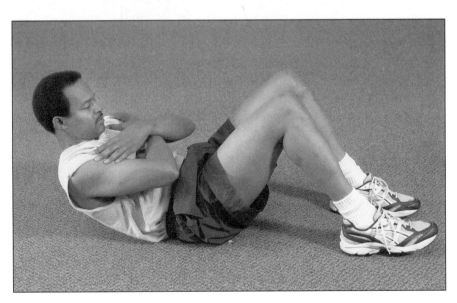

ROTATION CRUNCHES

Works the obliques

Lie on your back with your arms behind your head. Lift the upper body to touch each elbow to its opposite knee, making a twisting motion. Return to the original position. This exercise can be done with or without resistance.

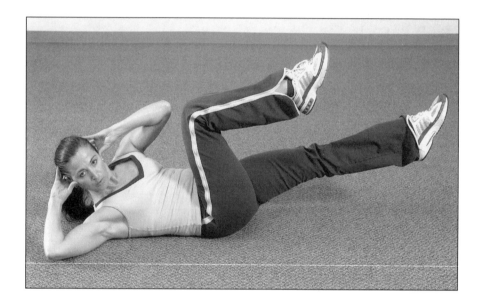

PULL-UPS (MACHINE)

Works the latissimus dorsi and teres major

Place your hands on the bar a bit farther than shoulder-width apart. Pull the body up using the arms until your head passes the level of the bar, then slowly return to the starting position.

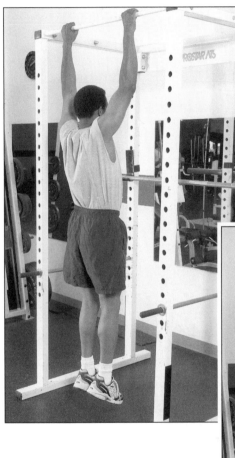

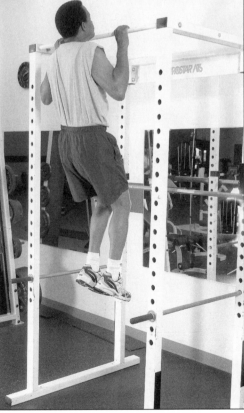

LAT PULLDOWNS (MACHINE)

Works the latissimus dorsi and teres major

Pull the bar down until it is level with the upper chest. Slowly let it return until the arms are completely extended.

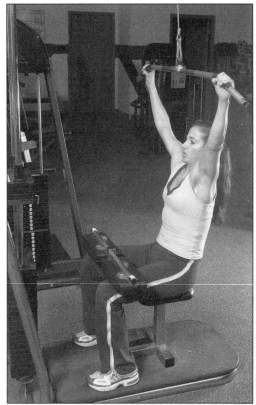

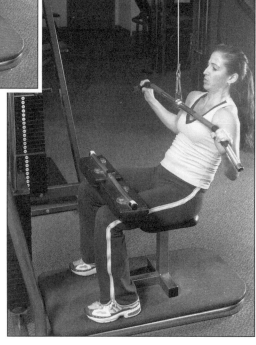

BENCH PRESS (MACHINE)

Works the pectoralis major

With hands shoulder-width apart, press upward until the arms are fully extended. Slowly return the weight until the chest is slightly stretched.

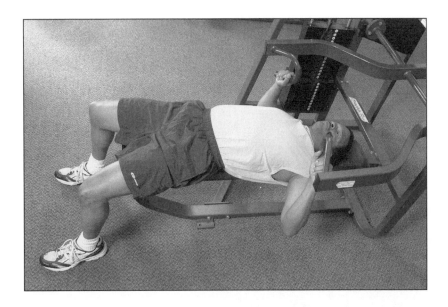

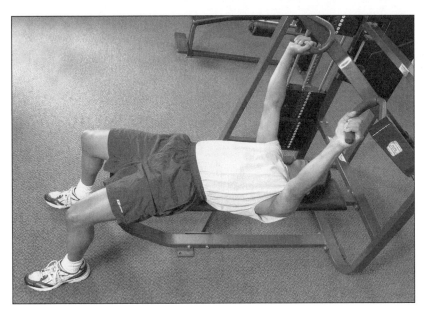

BUTTERFLY (MACHINE)

Works the pectoralis major

Place your forearms on the pads and push the pads together in front of the body. Return until the chest is slightly stretched.

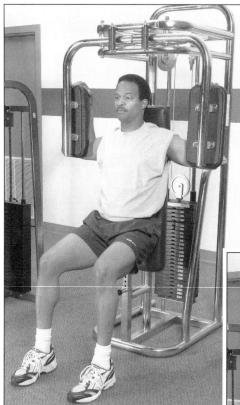

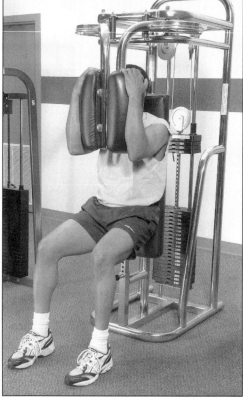

UPRIGHT ROWS

Works the back muscles

Hold a barbell with hands slightly wider than shoulder-width apart. Pull the barbell up to the level of the chest with the elbows leading and then slowly lower it back down. This exercise can also be done with dumbbells.

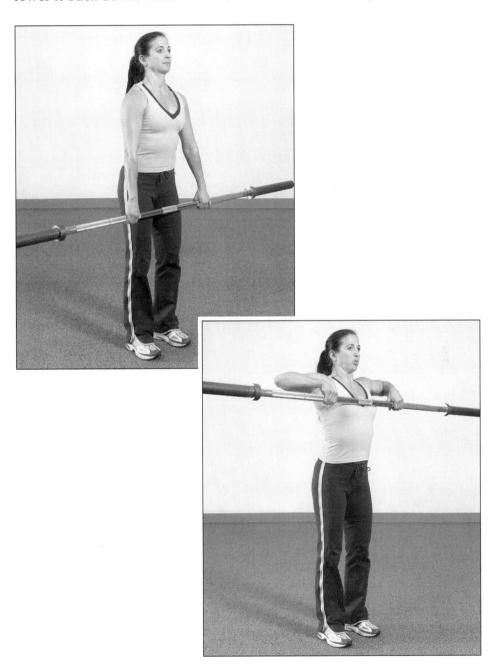

SHOULDER SHRUGS (BARBELL OR HAND WEIGHTS)

Works the upper trapezius

Grab the barbell and stand upright. Bring the barbell up as high as possible using the shoulder muscles (not arms) and then lower it.

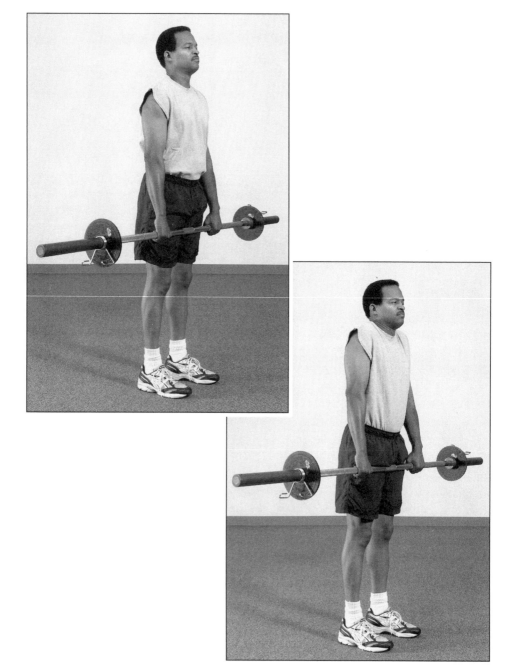

BICEPS CURLS (MACHINE OR HAND WEIGHTS)

Works the biceps brachii

With a dumbbell in each hand, start with your arms down at your sides and raise them by bending at the elbow until the hand weights are even with the shoulders. Lower the hand weights until the arms are fully extended.

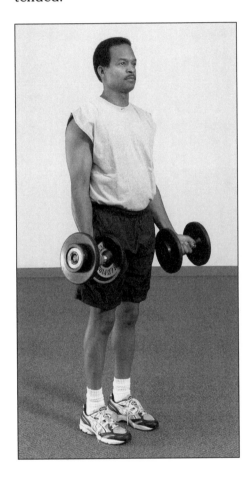
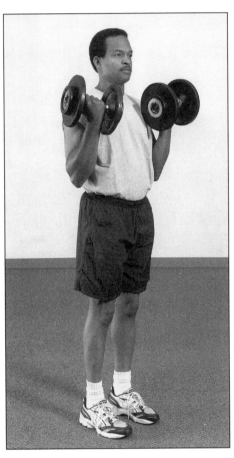

PREACHER CURLS (BENCH AND BARBELL)

Works the biceps brachii

Place your upper arms on the pad while seated on the bench. Raise the bar until the forearms are vertical, then slowly return the bar.

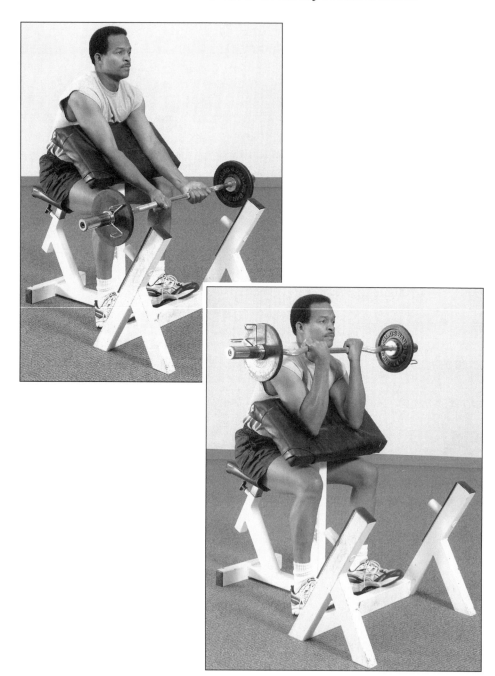

TRICEPS EXTENSIONS (HAND WEIGHTS)

Works the triceps brachii

Lower the dumbbell behind the head and keep the upper arms above the head. Raise the dumbbell above the head until the arms are almost fully extended.

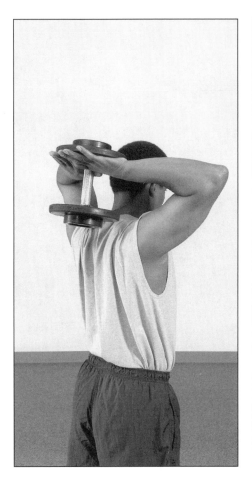
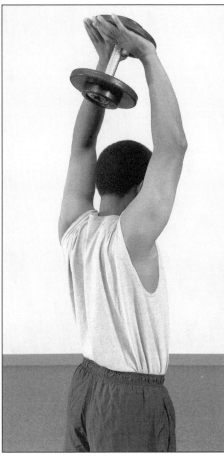

TRICEPS PUSHDOWN (MACHINE)

Works the triceps brachii

Start with the arms bent at a 90-degree angle, holding the cable about waist-high. Press downward until the arms are fully extended and return slowly to the start position.

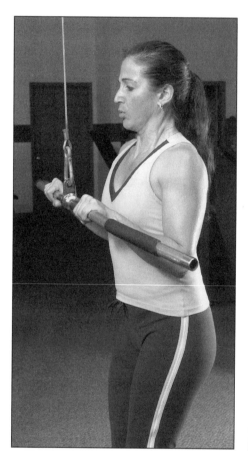
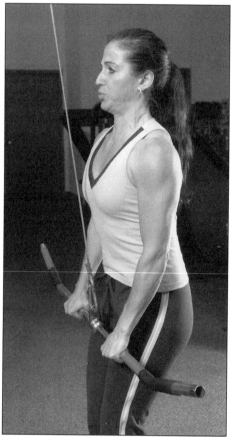

DIPS

Works the triceps brachii

Position yourself on a bench or chair with your feet on an object of similar height in front of you (for example, a stability ball). Slowly inch off the bench so that you are supporting yourself with your arms. Lower your body until the upper arms are parallel with the floor. Return to the start position. This exercise can also be done with the feet on the floor, as an easier option.

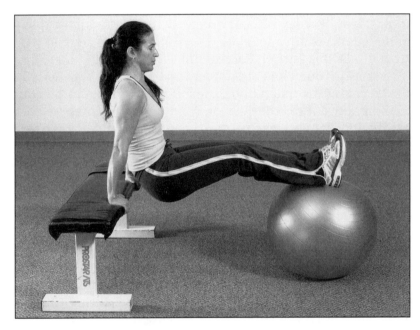

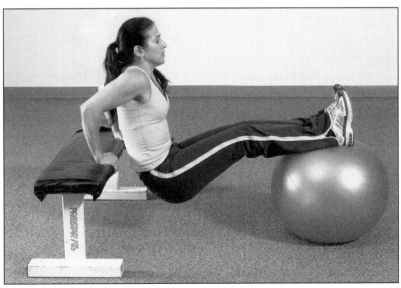

Overcoming Barriers to Exercise

In chapter 4 we discussed barriers to lifestyle changes. Because you are making lifestyle changes, it will be helpful now to figure what your potential barriers may be and then determine what you can do to overcome these barriers. One common roadblock that many people encounter is sometimes just not feeling up to exercising. That is a relatively easy barrier to overcome. First, remember that anyone can have days when for whatever reason you feel more fatigued and are just not up to exercising. One way to overcome this problem is to be prepared for it to happen. Instead of taking the day off and doing nothing (although when you're *really* fatigued this is not a bad idea), you should have several strategies ready to address this barrier. For example, the other day when I was getting ready to work out, I just did not feel up to doing what I had planned. So I cut the exercise session in half. Instead of running for 30 minutes, I ran for 15 minutes. After the session (and of course the best part—the shower), I felt great and was ready to continue my day knowing that I had gone ahead and done something good for my health, and that even though I did exercise, it was an easy exercise day, and because the exercise session was easy, I rested to some degree. In fact, after the exercise session, I felt invigorated. Thus, one strategy to overcome this barrier then is to do something rather than doing nothing.

Another barrier is not having time to exercise. In this case set aside a specific time in the day for your exercise session. You should make an appointment with yourself for a training session and write it in your daily schedule. Then make sure that you don't break the appointment with yourself. If someone asks to meet with you during this time period, your answer to this inquiry is that you already have something scheduled.

There are other strategies that you can use to help you overcome these barriers. For example, you could exercise with a friend. Having the responsibility of meeting and exercising with someone else is helpful. Another idea for overcoming barriers is to keep a physical activity or exercise journal. For some people, keeping track of what they do is excellent positive reinforcement. Give some thought as to what your barriers might be, and then plan ways to overcome these barriers.

Summary

Finding ways to increase your daily physical activity and implementing a cardiovascular and muscular fitness program will yield many health benefits, including positively altering your blood lipid and lipoprotein profile. Information presented in this chapter includes recommendations for increasing daily physical activities and specific guidelines for developing planned cardiovascular fitness and muscular fitness programs. In chapter 3, we discussed the concept that small increases in physical activity result in health benefits. However, in order to attain positive changes in your blood lipid and lipoprotein profile, you will need to develop a combined physical activity and planned exercise program resulting in energy expenditure of 1,200 to 1,500 kcal each week. This equals approximately 250 kcal of daily energy expenditure, which translates to about four or five hours of weekly physical activity and planned exercise.

ACTION PLAN:

BUILDING AN EXERCISE PROGRAM

- ☐ Know the distinctions between light, moderate, and vigorous physical activity.
- ☐ Set short- and long-term goals for physical activity and cardiovascular and muscular fitness.
- ☐ Find ways to incorporate physical activity into your daily life; for example, park far away from your building and walk.
- ☐ Understand the key exercise principles of overload, progression, specificity, and reversibility.
- ☐ Plan your cardiovascular exercise program to include the optimal amounts of exercise to lower cholesterol:
  - Frequency: three to five times per week
  - Intensity: 40 to 70 percent of HRmax
  - Duration: At least 30 minutes
- ☐ Use the equation (220 – age) to determine your maximum heart rate, and become familiar with the methods of measuring intensity.
- ☐ Make sure you know proper form for resistance training, and use the exercise descriptions and photos provided in this chapter to ensure you are keeping to that form.
- ☐ Use the sample exercise programs as they are, or adapt them to fit your preferences and needs.

CHAPTER 6

ESTABLISHING A HEART-HEALTHY DIET

Can you do without food? The obvious answer is no. In addition to being necessary for survival, food is at the center of social and family gatherings and has crept into our lives to meet emotional, social, and cultural needs. Food is used in place of speaking when words cannot be found and it is used to show love, sympathy, and friendship. In times of restlessness, boredom, or loneliness, food is often used for consolation. The connection between food and good feelings goes all the way back to babyhood when a full stomach was connected to feelings of joy, comfort, and safety. Our society's passionate relationship with food is complicated and at best difficult to untangle. Changing your dietary patterns to prevent, stop, or even reverse heart disease is going to present a challenge much like the challenge many people find in starting an exercise program. In general Americans consume too many calories and eat too much fat and sugar. We have developed these habits over many years, and they are a reflection of how we spend our coffee breaks, prepare our meals, and eat at fast-food restaurants. The suggestions offered in chapter 4 for making behavioral changes in developing an exercise program can also be helpful as you examine your patterns of food consumption.

From a dietary perspective the best way to positively affect blood cholesterol and the cholesterol associated with lipoproteins is to reduce body weight. This can be accomplished by lowering consumption of saturated fat and overall calories. In this chapter you will be introduced to topics including the changing face of food consumption in America, following a heart-healthy diet, and reducing saturated fat in your diet.

Food Consumption in the United States

Chapter 5 discussed adding more physical activity to your daily routine and developing a planned exercise program. One exercise not mentioned in chapter 5 is an exercise that should be completed during each meal: the "push-away." This exercise is very easy to do. You simply push away from the table. The gist of the push-away exercise is to get away from the table and not take additional portions. At the same time you are doing the push-away, you need to also be eating smaller portions. By doing the push-away and by eating smaller portions, you eat less during a meal and reduce the amount of calories consumed. Most Americans eat much more food than they really need. While doing a push-away, here are some thoughts to keep in mind. As you eat a meal, you might feel that you are not yet satisfied and need to eat a second or a third serving. However, the brain may take 15 minutes or more to realize that the stomach is getting full. Try eating slowly, eating smaller portion sizes, and allowing more time for your digestive system and your brain to communicate. In this way you allow your brain to catch up with your stomach. Also, consider eating a smaller first serving. Many people have already adjusted their eating habits by not eating a second or third serving, but these same people will eat an extraordinarily large first portion. Keeping your portions small is important.

Let's turn our focus to some interesting eating trends found in America and how our dietary habits have changed in the last 50 years. Americans of the 21st century consume several hundred more calories per day than Americans in previous decades. Today the average American eats approximately 2,700 calories each day, which is 500 calories above the average in 1970 and 700 calories above the average in the late 1950s. In addition, when Americans began to eat more, they also began to exercise less.

Another interesting trend is that Americans are eating out more often. When dining out, people consume much more food than they need and eat foods that are high in calories. These behaviors have helped make weight gain a national problem. Weight gain is responsible for greater incidence of obesity, and obesity is a major health concern because it increases the occurrence of associated chronic diseases like heart disease, diabetes, and cancer. Excessive food consumption is also associated with elevated levels of blood cholesterol, triglycerides, and LDL-C. Fortunately, by lowering caloric consumption and fat intake, you can reduce body weight. This behavior change has an enormous positive effect on your blood cholesterol and triglyceride levels as well as your LDL-C.

Building a Heart-Healthy Diet

As you consider starting to eat a heart-healthy diet, one of the things to think about is eating a proper mix of carbohydrate, protein, and fat. Heart-healthy eating patterns include consuming a variety of fruits, vegetables, grains, low-fat or nonfat dairy products, fish, legumes (beans), poultry, and lean meats. Most health professionals working in disease prevention recommend a nutritional diet that contains approximately 50 to 60 percent carbohydrate and 12 to 15 percent protein. No more than 30 percent of the calories should come from fat.

Most people have heard the recommendation to eat a low-fat, low-cholesterol diet. While it's true that dietary cholesterol is linked to heart disease, a greater concern is the cholesterol produced by the body. Surprisingly, the amount of cholesterol in food is not very strongly linked to blood cholesterol levels. Instead, dietary saturated fat is the problem, as it has the biggest influence on blood cholesterol levels and increases the risk for certain diseases. The key to altering blood cholesterol through dietary fat is to substitute healthy fat for unhealthy fat. Many health agencies, including the American Dietetic Association, American Diabetes Association, and American Heart Association, recommend limiting fat intake to no more than 30 percent of total daily calories to prevent disease. For adults with heart disease, a diet where no more than 20 percent of calories comes from fat is wise. In this chapter, you will learn about the various forms of dietary fat and their effects on blood cholesterol, the cholesterol associated with blood lipoproteins, and the other nutrients that play a part in a healthy diet.

Carbohydrate

Carbohydrate is mainly sugar and starch produced by plants. Along with fat and protein, carbohydrate makes up one of the three types of nutrients that the body uses as an energy source. One gram of carbohydrate equals four energy calories. Carbohydrate is found in simple forms, or *simple carbohydrate,* such as sugars, and in complex forms or *complex carbohydrate,* such as starch and fiber. Simple carbohydrate and complex carbohydrate (except for fiber) are both broken down by the body into glucose to be used for energy.

Several forms of simple carbohydrate exist. One is sucrose, also referred to as table sugar, which is found in most candies and is associated with higher blood triglyceride and total cholesterol levels and lower blood HDL-C levels. Another simple sugar is *fructose,* which is found in fruit. Fructose is a much healthier sugar than sucrose because it produces a slower rise in blood sugar; because of this fact, fructose provides some advantages for people with diabetes. As with any sugar, however, excess consumption of fructose is associated with elevated blood triglyceride and total cholesterol levels and lower HDL-C levels.

Complex carbohydrate includes starches and fibers. The complex carbohydrate found in whole grains, vegetables, and brown rice is preferred over refined starches such as those found in pasta, white rice, and white-flour products. Dietary intake of complex carbohydrate can lower blood cholesterol when it is substituted for saturated fat. Complex carbohydrate can be found in a variety of foods, such as brown or wild rice, cereals, dried fruit, bran, whole grains, oats, breads, pastas, and legumes—some of the healthiest foods on the planet. Complex carbohydrate is also a form of low-glycemic food. This means that digestion takes place more slowly, causing a slower, much gentler rise in blood sugar. In contrast to high-glycemic carbohydrate (i.e., table sugar, candy, syrup, honey), low-glycemic carbohydrate is associated with lower heart disease risk and it helps control type 2 diabetes. Overall, foods high in complex carbohydrate are full of nutrients, vitamins, minerals, fiber, and antioxidants and are an important part of a healthy diet.

Fiber

Fiber refers to plant materials that we cannot digest. Our bodies do not have the necessary enzymes to break fiber down so that it can be digested and absorbed. Fiber promotes health by reducing the risk for chronic conditions like constipation, hemorrhoids, and diverticulosis (a condition in which pouches develop in the large intestine and can become inflamed). Fiber is also linked to reduced risk for some cancers, especially colon and breast cancer. Further, a diet rich in fiber may lower total blood cholesterol and LDL-C, thereby reducing risk of heart disease. Fiber also helps to lower blood sugar and manage diabetes. Fiber is found in two forms, soluble and insoluble. *Soluble fiber* can mix with water while *insoluble fiber* absorbs water and provides bulk. Food sources of soluble fiber are oat products and oat bran, dried beans and peas, barley, fruits like oranges and apples, and vegetables such as carrots. Food sources of insoluble fiber include whole-wheat products; wheat bran; flaxseed; vegetables such as green beans, cauliflower, and potato skins; and fruit skins and root vegetable skins.

Soluble fiber is more important than insoluble fiber in lowering total cholesterol and LDL-C and thereby reducing risk of heart disease. Soluble fiber is also important in regulating blood sugar for people with diabetes. Insoluble dietary fiber promotes regular bowel movement and enhances the removal of toxic waste at faster rates. This aids in keeping an optimal intestinal acid–base balance and prevents microbes from producing cancer substances. All of these actions reduce the risk of colon cancer.

Fiber is thought to lower blood cholesterol levels by attaching to cholesterol and other fats as they move through the intestine. The body cannot absorb fiber, so when cholesterol becomes attached to the fiber, neither the attached cholesterol nor the fiber can be absorbed. Both the fiber and the attached cholesterol will continue to move through the digestive system. Soluble fiber (5 to 10 grams per day) can help lower total cholesterol and LDL-C levels by as much as 25 percent. The Food and Drug Administration (FDA), the National Academy of Sciences (NAS), the U.S. Department of Agriculture (USDA), and the American Cancer Society (ACS) all recommend consuming 25 to 35 grams of fiber per day. Currently, most Americans eat less than 10 grams of fiber per day.

Protein

Protein should provide 12 to 15 percent of total calories consumed. One gram of protein contains four calories of energy, but only about 5 percent of dietary protein is used for energy. Most dietary protein is used for building and repairing tissue; thus protein is essential for developing strong muscles and bones. The best sources of protein are fish, poultry, and soy, and you should restrict your dietary intake of red meat or any meat that is not lean.

Fish

Fish is likely the best source of protein. Choose fish that are not grown on farms, because they have fewer nutrients (e.g., omega-3 fatty acids). The way to gain the most heart-healthy benefits from fish is to eat salmon, mackerel, sardines, halibut, and tuna. These types of fish are also high in omega-3 fatty acids (more on this fat later). By eating even moderate amounts of omega-3 fatty acids, you can lower blood triglyceride levels with an added benefit of lowering the tendency of the blood to clot. While eating fish only once a week is associated with a lower risk of heart attack, five or six weekly servings of fish may increase the risk of stroke. Also, consuming large amounts of certain fish, such as tuna, may increase the risk of mercury toxicity.

Soy

Soy is an excellent food because it contains both soluble and insoluble fiber, omega-3 fatty acids (see the section on dietary fat), and provides all essential proteins. One nutrient found in soy is a natural estrogen called *isoflavones,* which have positive effects on lipid levels. Recent research suggests that soy's proteins lower blood total cholesterol, LDL-C, and triglyceride levels. Daily consumption of an average of 47 grams of soy protein decreased total cholesterol by 9 percent, decreased LDL-cholesterol by 12 percent, decreased triglycerides by 11 percent, and increased HDL-cholesterol by 3 percent. One possible concern about high soy intake is its potential to adversely affect the fetus during pregnancy due to soy's high amounts of natural estrogen. Also, women with estrogen-sensitive cancers or a family history of such cancers should be aware that soy contains *phytoestrogens*, which may further increase cancer risk. However, before any further conclusions can be stated more research in this area is needed.

Beef, Poultry, and Pork

The problem with beef is not the meat itself. The problem is its fat content. To protect your heart, you should choose fish or poultry over beef or pork. Beef is more acceptable when its saturated fat is low (saturated fat found in meat is the primary danger to the heart). The fat content of meat varies and depends on the type of meat and cut. For best results in lowering blood cholesterol, eat skinless chicken or turkey. However, the leanest cuts of pork (loin and tenderloin), veal, and beef are nearly comparable to chicken in calories and fat content. Lean beef, pork, and chicken have similar effects on lowering blood total cholesterol and LDL-C levels. However, fish positively affects blood cholesterol more than chicken and lean beef do. For the best heart health, fish is a more desirable choice.

Dietary Fat

Dietary fat is a major source of calories and improves the taste of foods. Fat provides nine calories per fat gram, more than twice the number of calories provided by carbohydrate or protein. Fat does have important functions. It is essential in the formation of body structures such as muscles, nerves, membranes, and blood vessels, and it aids in the proper absorption of fat-soluble vitamins A, D, E, and K. In general, dietary fat that originates from animals is referred to as saturated fat, and fat that originates from vegetables is referred to as unsaturated fat, with the exception of coconut, coconut oil, palm oil, and palm kernel oil.

In the last 50 years as Americans have consumed more food, they have also consumed a greater amount of dietary fat, including saturated or animal fat. Saturated fat has many harmful effects, but perhaps the most important damaging effect is the impairment of the liver's ability to remove cholesterol from the blood. As a result, blood cholesterol and LDL-C levels become elevated.

Cholesterol

Cholesterol is found in all animal products, including beef, poultry, seafood, eggs, and dairy products such as cheese and milk. Egg yolks and organ meats like liver, brains, and kidneys are especially high in cholesterol. The NCEP recommends eating less than 300 milligrams of dietary cholesterol each day.

Saturated Fat

Saturated fat is found mainly in animal fats and to a lesser extent in seafood, whole-milk dairy products, and poultry skin. A few plant foods are also high in saturated fat (coconut, coconut oil, palm oil, and palm kernel oil). Saturated fat is solid at room temperatures. Diets rich in saturated fat can raise blood total cholesterol and LDL-C levels more than dietary cholesterol.

Trans Fat

Trans-fatty acids, or trans fat, are produced by a manufacturing process. This process is achieved by heating liquid vegetable oils in the presence of hydrogen, creating hydrogenated oil. The more hydrogenated an oil is, the harder the fat becomes at room temperature. Trans fat exists in many commercially prepared foods, such as baked goods, margarine, snacks, and most other processed foods. Commercially prepared fast foods, like french fries and onion rings, also contain a good deal of trans fat. Trans fat is worse than saturated fat because it has a greater tendency to raise blood cholesterol and LDL-C levels while lowering HDL-C levels.

As awareness about trans fat increases, more trans fat–free products are becoming available. Labeling of trans-fat content has long been up to the manufacturer's discretion. However, a recent report on trans fat from the Institute of Medicine concluded that there is no safe level of dietary trans fat. This proclamation finally prompted the FDA to require that trans fat be listed as part of the nutrition facts food label. But until labels that include trans fat begin to appear, you need to read labels closely to determine if a processed food contains trans fat. Check the ingredient list for hydrogenated oils or partially hydrogenated oils. The higher up on this list the hydrogenated items appear, the greater the trans-fat content in the product.

Unsaturated Fat

Some fats are healthy because they lower blood cholesterol levels. One type of these fats is referred to as unsaturated fat. Unsaturated fat is found in products derived from plant sources (vegetable oils, nuts, and seeds). The two main categories are *monounsaturated fats* and *polyunsaturated fats.*

Monounsaturated fats remain liquid at low temperatures and are found in vegetable oils such as olive, canola, and peanut oils. This fat can lower blood cholesterol and LDL-C without altering HDL-C. On the other hand, too much dietary monounsaturated fat will cause excessive body fat and even elevated blood cholesterol.

Polyunsaturated fats are found in sunflower, corn, and soybean oils and are also present in fish and fish oils. These fats are generally liquid at room temperature. Dietary polyunsaturated fats lower blood triglyceride, total cholesterol, and LDL-C levels, but they also lower HDL-C levels. Thus, while both monounsaturated and polyunsaturated are considered healthy, you should follow recommended guidelines and limit your consumption of these types of fat. For a diet of 2,000 calories per day, roughly 5.5 to 9 percent of those calories should come from polyunsaturated fat and 10 to 11 percent from monounsaturated fat.

Because monounsaturated and polyunsaturated fats in proper amounts can result in positive changes in blood lipids and lipoproteins, they are referred to as healthy fats. In the Nurses' Health Study (NHS), Harvard researchers found that replacing 80 calories of carbohydrate with 80 calories of either polyunsaturated or monounsaturated fat lowered the risk for heart disease by about 30 to 40 percent (Hu, Manson, and Willett 2001).

Omega-3 Fatty Acids

Fish is an important source of the polyunsaturated fat known as omega-3 fatty acids. This type of fat has received much attention for its potential in lowering risk of heart disease. Omega-3 fatty acids seem to raise HDL-C levels and make blood platelets less likely to clot. Both of these benefits reduce the likelihood of a heart attack. Salmon, albacore tuna, mackerel, sardines, herring, and rainbow trout all have high amounts of omega-3 fatty acids. Although scientists do not completely understand how omega-3 fatty acids work in disease prevention, adding these types of fish to the diet may help protect you from heart disease, and there are no known risks. The American Heart Association currently recommends that everyone eat at least two servings of these types of fish a week.

Investigating Diet Plans

You can take many different dietary approaches in lowering your blood cholesterol. The USDA started publishing *A Pattern for Daily Food Choices* in the 1980s. The Food Guide Pyramid was first released in 1992. The Nutrition Labeling and Education Act placed a nutrition label on every product, making it easier for people to follow the pyramid's guidelines. Many new diets are constantly emerging with miraculous claims, making it a struggle for Americans to follow the guidelines from the USDA.

In 2005, the USDA released their new dietary guidelines. These guidelines provide essential strategies for eating a heart-healthy diet (see table 6.1). By focusing on these guidelines, you will be better able to achieve and maintain a healthy body weight through healthier food choices and dietary practices. In this section we discuss some diet plans that can help you develop healthy eating habits that follow the USDA guidelines.

Table 6.1   USDA Dietary Guidelines

Grains	Vegetables	Fruits	Milk	Meat and beans
Eat at least 3 oz of whole-grain cereals, breads, crackers, rice, or pasta every day. 1 oz is about 1 slice of bread, 1 cup of breakfast cereal, or ½ cup of cooked rice, cereal, or pasta.	Eat more dark-green vegetables like broccoli, spinach, and other dark leafy greens. Eat more orange vegetables like carrots and sweet potatoes. Eat more dry beans and peas like pinto beans, kidney beans, and lentils.	Eat a variety of fruits. Choose fresh, frozen, canned, or dried fruit. Go easy on fruit juices.	Choose low-fat or fat-free milk, yogurt, and other milk products. If you don't or can't consume milk, choose lactose-free products or other calcium sources such as fortified foods and beverages.	Choose low-fat or lean meats and poultry. Bake it, broil it, or grill it. Vary your protein routine— choose more fish, beans, peas, nuts, and seeds.
For a 2,000-calorie diet, you need the following amounts from each food group. To find the amounts that are right for you, go to http://MyPyramid.gov.				
Eat 6 oz every day.	Eat 2½ cups every day.	Eat 2 cups every day.	Eat 3 cups every day (2 cups for kids aged 2 to 8).	Eat 5½ oz every day.

Find your balance between food and physical activity.

- Be sure to stay within your daily calorie needs.
- Be physically active for at least 30 minutes most days of the week.
- About 60 minutes a day of physical activity may be needed to prevent weight gain.
- For sustaining weight loss, at least 60 to 90 minutes a day of physical activity may be required.
- Children and teenagers should be physically active for 60 minutes most days.

Know the limits on fats, sugars, and salt (sodium).

- Consume most of your fat from fish, nuts, and vegetable oils.
- Limit solid fats like butter, margarine, shortening, and lard as well as foods that contain these fats.
- Check the nutrition label to keep saturated fats, trans fats, and sodium low.
- Choose food and beverages low in added sugars. Added sugars contribute calories with few, if any, nutrients.

From the US Department of Agriculture, Center for Nutrition Policy and Promotion.

5 A Day for Better Health

The 5 A Day campaign is a national program designed to teach Americans about the importance of including at least five servings of fruits and vegetables in their daily diets. Fruits and vegetables contain vitamins, minerals, fiber, and disease-fighting phytochemicals that are necessary for promoting good health and reducing risk of certain diseases. By eating five or more servings of fruits and vegetables every day, you are well on your way to reducing your risk of heart disease, high blood pressure, type 2 diabetes, and certain cancers. This reduction in risk is easily achieved by choosing a wide variety of colorful vegetables and fruit every day as part of a meal or as healthy snacks. The 5 A Day program is an easy way to track your dietary intake of fresh fruit and vegetables and to set goals to achieve healthy dietary habits.

The program involves five groups of fruits and vegetables categorized by color. All five of these color groups are associated with certain phytochemicals. Eating food from each color group promotes the healthy functioning of different body systems. The blue and purple group is full of health-promoting nutrients that help maintain urinary tract health and memory function and reduce the risk of developing some cancers. Some common foods in this group are blackberries, blueberries, eggplants, and plums. The green group contains antioxidants (substances such as vitamin E and vitamin C that are thought to protect body cells from damaging effects of metabolism). Foods in the green group help protect vision from deterioration and promote bone and teeth development. They also can help reduce the risk for some cancers. Green apples, kiwis, green grapes, broccoli, green beans, and leafy greens are just some of the many foods in the green group. The white group has phytochemicals that promote a healthy heart, a lower risk of some cancers, and HDL-C. Onions, bananas, cauliflower, and dates are some of the foods in the white group. The yellow and orange group includes items such as cantaloupe, oranges, pineapples, sweet corn, carrots, and yellow peppers. These foods have nutrients that help keep the immune system healthy while also protecting vision, promoting heart health, and reducing the risk for some cancers. Foods in the red group include red apples, cranberries, strawberries, tomatoes, red potatoes, and beets. These are just some of the foods you can choose from to help promote heart health, memory function, urinary-tract health, and a lower risk for some cancers.

For more information on each of the color groups, visit www.5aday.com/html/colorway/colorway_home.php. You can also find a table containing an extensive list of fruits and vegetables along with their amounts of calories, fiber, vitamin A, vitamin C, potassium, and folate at www.dole5aday.com/ReferenceCenter/NutritionCenter/Chart/R_NutrChart.jsp.

Therapeutic Lifestyle Changes (TLC)

People who have high blood cholesterol and high LDL-C or who have known cardiovascular disease should adopt the Therapeutic Lifestyle Changes (TLC) diet. In May 2001, the NCEP released their new guidelines for cholesterol management in the *Third Report of the Expert Panel on Detection, Evaluation, and Treatment of High Blood Cholesterol in Adults.* This report recognized that the best way to lower your blood cholesterol level is to eat less saturated fat and cholesterol and to control your weight. Here are some basic dietary recommendations.

- Total calories should be adjusted to help you reach and maintain a healthy body weight.
- Saturated fat intake should be no more than 10 percent of total calories.
- Polyunsaturated fat intake can be up to 10 percent of calories.
- Monounsaturated fat can be up to 15 percent of total calories.
- Total dietary fat intake should be adjusted to caloric needs. Over-weight people should consume no more than 30 percent of total calories from fat.
- Dietary cholesterol intake should be less than 300 milligrams per day.
- Sodium consumption should be less than 2,400 milligrams per day, or about one teaspoon of sodium chloride (salt).

For more tips on incorporating these healthy eating guidelines, see the following sidebar.

Healthy Food Choices

- Eat plenty of fresh fruits and vegetables rather than the juice forms of the same vegetables.
- Eat the skin of clean fruits and vegetables.
- Eat bran and whole-grain cereals and breads.
- As you consume more fiber, drink more water.
- Eat plenty of fresh food rather than processed food.
- Get fiber from foods instead of from supplements because foods are more nutritious.
- Eat more legumes (red, black, pinto, and garbanzo beans) and dishes made with them, such as hummus.
- The fat in dairy foods is mostly saturated. Try nonfat or low-fat versions.

DASH Diet

The DASH diet (Dietary Approaches to Stop Hypertension) is rich in vegetables and fruit and low in fat and cholesterol. The fruits and vegetables in the DASH eating plan are higher in fiber and lower in sucrose (see the following sidebar for information on how many fruits and vegetables to eat in a day). Scientists have found that the DASH diet significantly reduces the levels of total cholesterol and LDL-C. When compared to persons not on any particular diet, individuals on the DASH diet on average reduced their levels of blood cholesterol by 7 percent and their levels of blood LDL-C by 9 percent. Blood triglyceride levels, which also increase risk of heart disease, were not significantly changed in participants on the DASH diet, but blood HDL-C levels decreased by about 8 percent. The HDL-C drop is directly related to the person's prediet HDL-C level. Thus, when using the DASH diet, blood HDL-C levels could decrease, most likely in people who have higher HDL levels to begin with. In addition, the DASH eating plan lowers the level of homocysteine, an amino acid that has been related to risk of heart disease. See table 6.2 for a description of the recommendations for the DASH diet.

A Day's Dose of Fruits and Vegetables

This is not a complete meal plan because it does not include meat, grains, dairy products, or fat. It just gives an idea of how many fruits and vegetables to include in your daily meals according to the DASH diet.

Breakfast: Have 3/4 cup of 100 percent orange juice, and put 1/2 cup of fresh blueberries on whole-grain cereal.

Snack: Slice a banana onto whole-wheat bread with peanut butter.

Lunch: Combine 2 cups of diced tomatoes, 2 cups of diced cucumbers, and 2 cups of leafy green lettuce (not iceberg) or spinach.

Dinner: Serve two baked sweet potatoes and 2 cups of peas (frozen or fresh) with dinner.

Mediterranean Diet

The incidence of heart disease among people in the Mediterranean region is quite lower than that found in many other places in the world. Much of this difference has been attributed to what has been termed the Mediterranean diet. At least 16 countries that border the Mediterranean Sea and have differences in cultures, ethnic backgrounds, religions, economies, and agricultural production contribute to the Mediterranean diet. These different groups of people have varying eating patterns between countries and even differences between regions within a country. Although many cultural and dietary differences exist and no single

Table 6.2   The DASH Diet

Food group	Daily servings	Serving sizes	Examples and notes	Significance to the DASH eating plan
Grains and grain products	7–8	1 slice bread; 1 oz dry cereal;* 1/2 cup cooked cereals, rice, or pasta	Whole-wheat bread, English muffin, pita bread, bagel, cereals, grits, oatmeal, crackers, unsalted pretzels and popcorn	Major sources of energy and fiber
Vegetables	4–5	1 cup raw leafy vegetables, 1/2 cup cooked vegetables, 6 oz (150 ml) vegetable juice	Tomatoes, potatoes, carrots, peas, squash, broccoli, turnip greens, collards, kale, spinach, artichokes, green beans, lima beans, sweet potatoes	Rich sources of potassium, magnesium, and fiber
Fruits	4–5	1 medium fruit; 1/4 cup dried fruit; 1/2 cup fresh, frozen, or canned fruit; 6 oz (150 ml) fruit juice	Apricots, bananas, dates, grapes, oranges, orange juice, grapefruit, mangoes, melons, peaches, pineapples, prunes, raisins, strawberries, tangerines	Important sources of potassium, magnesium, and fiber
Low-fat or nonfat dairy foods	2–3	8 oz (200 ml) milk, 1 cup yogurt, 1.5 oz (40 g) cheese	Skim or semiskim milk, nonfat or low-fat frozen yogurt, nonfat or low-fat cheese	Major sources of calcium and protein
Meats, poultry, and fish	2 or less	3 oz (80 g) cooked meat, poultry, or fish	Lean cuts with visible fat trimmed away; broiled, roasted, boiled instead of fried; skin removed from poultry	Rich sources of protein and magnesium
Nuts, seeds, and dry beans	4–5 per week	1.5 oz or 1/3 cup nuts, 2 tbsp or .5 oz seeds, 1/2 cup cooked dry beans	Almonds, mixed nuts, peanuts, sunflower seeds, kidney beans, lentils	Rich sources of energy, magnesium, potassium, protein, and fiber
Fats and oils**	2–3	1 tsp soft margarine, 1 tbsp low-fat mayonnaise, 2 tbsp light salad dressing, 1 tsp vegetable oil	Soft margarine, low-fat mayonnaise, light salad dressing, vegetable oil (such as olive, corn, canola, or safflower)	DASH has 27 percent of calories as fat, including fat in or added to foods
Sweets	5	1 tbsp sugar, 1 tbsp jelly or jam, .5 oz jelly beans, 8 oz lemonade	Maple syrup, sugar, jelly, jam, fruit-flavored gelatin, jelly beans, hard candy, fruit punch, sorbet, ices	Sweets should be low in fat

*Equals 1/2 to 1 1/4 cups, depending on cereal type. Check the product's Nutrition Facts Label.
**Fat content changes serving counts for fats and oils: For example, 1 tbsp of regular salad dressing equals 1 serving; 1 tbsp of a low-fat dressing equals 1/2 serving; 1 tbsp of a nonfat dressing equals 0 servings.

From the National Heart, Lung and Blood Institute and the National Institutes of Health (NIH), a section of the US Department of Health and Human Services. www.nhlbi.nih.gov/health/public/heart/hbp/dash/new_dash.pdf

Mediterranean diet exists, Mediterranean dietary patterns have these common characteristics:

- A great deal of fruits, vegetables, bread and other cereals, potatoes, beans, nuts, and seeds are consumed.
- Olive oil is used as an important source of monounsaturated fat.
- Dairy products, fish, and poultry are consumed in low to moderate amounts, and little red meat is eaten.
- Eggs are consumed no more than four times a week.
- Red wine is consumed in low to moderate amounts.

The Mediterranean diet is similar to the TLC dietary guidelines in some respects. In general, the diets of Mediterranean people contain a relatively high percentage of calories from fat. This fact is perhaps one reason why there are increasing rates of obesity in Mediterranean countries. However, people who follow the average Mediterranean diet eat less saturated fat than those who eat the average American diet. In fact, consumption of saturated fat in the Mediterranean diet is well within TLC dietary guidelines. More than half of the fat calories in a Mediterranean diet come from monounsaturated fat (mainly from olive oil). The difference is that consumption of monounsaturated fat does not raise blood cholesterol levels the way consumption of saturated fat does. See table 6.3 for a summary of the recommendations of the Mediterranean diet.

Table 6.3   *Recommendations for the Mediterranean Diet*

Frequency	Daily	Weekly	Monthly
Foods (in order of relative amount; see following note)	Bread, pasta, rice, couscous, polenta, other whole grains, potatoes Fruits Beans, legumes, nuts Vegetables Olive oil Cheese, yogurt	Fish Poultry Eggs Sweets	Meat

Created from information from the Mediterranean diet pyramid, from Willet et al., 1995, "Mediterranean diet pyramid: A cultural model for healthy eating," *American Journal of Clinical Nutrition* 61:1402S-1406S. Foods are listed in order of their placement in the pyramid from the bottom up. For example, among the daily foods, breads, pasta, rice, and so on are in the widest part of the pyramid, while cheese and yogurt are in the narrowest part of the pyramid.

Overcoming Barriers to Successful Dietary Changes

We have discussed barriers that keep us from successfully changing behavior. Just as barriers exist for beginning and maintaining a regular exercise and physical activity program, similar barriers exist for making successful dietary changes. Here are a few ideas to keep in mind as you start developing heart-healthy eating patterns.

• *Eating only as much as you need.* Remember to do the push-away and to reduce your serving sizes. By reducing the total number of calories you consume, you are starting a lifestyle change that can lead to lower body weight and lower blood cholesterol.

• *Eating out.* When dining out, ask for a heart-healthy menu. Also, look at the portion sizes. You can reduce your caloric intake by not eating all that is served or by dividing the portion in half and taking the remainder home for a later meal.

• *Eating slowly.* By eating slowly you give your brain more time to recognize how much you have eaten and how full your stomach is. This technique works very closely with the push-away.

• *Keeping track of what you eat.* Many people find that knowing how much they are eating is helpful in reducing the amount they consume. Keep a record of all that you eat for several days, and then review this record and develop strategies for exchanging some foods for other foods and eliminating some foods altogether. Periodically keep a record of what you eat and reassess your eating habits. This would be a good time to visit a dietitian and get advice.

Finally, you may encounter situations where you fall off the wagon. One time of not following proper dietary recommendations does not equal the end of your dietary behavior change. If you follow a heart-healthy diet all the time, it is not going to hurt you to occasionally fall off the wagon, but do not let one time lead to a series of "one-time" negative behaviors. Rather, consider each situation as its own challenge. Find a way to make the best of the circumstances and overcome the setting as you develop and maintain heart-healthy behaviors. When you fall off the wagon, get right back on.

The appendix beginning on page 161 contains several recipes for dishes that follow the principles of healthy eating. You can use these recipes for meal planning and even vary them slightly to fit your own tastes.

Healthy Diet Resources

Here are some Web sites that you may find helpful in your quest for a well-balanced, heart-healthy diet:

www.well-connected.com/rreports/doc43full.html

http://health.allrefer.com/health/carbohydrates-complex-carbohydrates.html

http://health.allrefer.com/health/carbohydrates-simple-carbohydrates.html

www.healthcastle.com/fiber-solubleinsoluble.shtml

www.medterms.com/script/main/art.asp?articlekey=13977

www.wholehealthmd.com/refshelf/substances_view/1,1525,10057,00.html# Health_Benefits

www.teenhealthfx.com/answers/Sports/6009.html

www.heartcenteronline.com/myheartdr/common/artprn_rev.cfm?filename=& ARTID=355

www.guidofguida.it/MedDiet.htm

Summary

Developing healthy dietary behaviors is as important as developing regular exercise habits. Regular exercise and good eating behaviors work together to affect blood cholesterol. By following the NCEP recommendations of eating fresh fruits, vegetables, nuts (especially walnuts and almonds), and less saturated fat; keeping consumption of dairy products low to moderate; and reducing caloric intake, you can lower your body weight and reduce blood cholesterol, LDL-C, and triglyceride levels.

ACTION PLAN:

ESTABLISHING A HEART-HEALTHY DIET

- ☐ Identify the major food trends in the United States and know the negatives of these habits.
- ☐ Develop an understanding of the relationship between nutritional behavior and diseases like heart disease.
- ☐ Be familiar with the essential nutrients of carbohydrate, protein, fiber, and dietary fat; the foods that are significant sources of these nutrients; and the recommended levels of each nutrient.
- ☐ Identify strategies to alter present eating habits so that you consume less saturated and trans fat while consuming more fresh vegetables and fruits. Options include
  - the 5 A Day program,
  - Therapeutic Lifestyle Changes (TLC),
  - the DASH diet, and
  - the Mediterranean diet.
- ☐ Identify and overcome barriers to change in developing healthy eating plans.

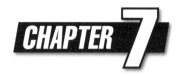
CHOOSING MEDICATION FOR LOWER CHOLESTEROL

The incidence of heart disease and related deaths is reduced when people who have high blood cholesterol follow appropriate lipid-lowering recommendations for exercise, diet, and medications. Exercise and diet lifestyle changes are important and you should exhaust every avenue in terms of changing your diet and exercise habits to positively affect blood cholesterol and lipoproteins. The first course of action in reducing your blood cholesterol and LDL-C is to start an exercise program and begin following a heart-healthy diet. These measures are effective for most people in moving high blood cholesterol toward acceptable levels.

Despite your best efforts, though, sometimes exercise, diet, and weight-loss programs are not enough to lower your blood cholesterol levels. Unfortunately, while changing your way of living plays an important role in positively influencing your cholesterol level, these changes alone are not the only factors that contribute to high blood cholesterol. For some individuals, the liver simply produces too much cholesterol. If this is the case, a heart-healthy diet and increased physical activity and planned exercise still provide many health benefits and should be continued, but without the aid of lipid-lowering medications, your blood cholesterol is not likely to reach desirable levels.

If your blood cholesterol and LDL-C are still elevated after three to six months of starting exercise and diet therapeutic lifestyle programs, if you are genetically predisposed to having high cholesterol, or if you are having difficulty losing weight, there are many medications available for managing cholesterol. Having your physician prescribe medications does not mean that you have failed; it only means that you need extra assistance in order to meet your cholesterol goals.

Starting a lipid-lowering drug is not a free pass to return to your old lifestyle. If you continue to follow a heart-healthy diet and get plenty of exercise, your doctor will likely prescribe the lowest dose possible of lipid-lowering medications. In fact, most people taking cholesterol medication alone do not always reach their blood cholesterol goals. You are more likely to lower your blood cholesterol and LDL-C levels if you exercise regularly, eat a heart-healthy diet, and take your medications.

While taking lipid-lowering medications, you can greatly reduce your risk of having a heart attack or needing bypass surgery, though drug therapy must continue for at least one year before a substantial decrease in the risk of death or illness due to heart disease is noticed. What you may not realize is that once you start a lipid-lowering medication, you are committed to medication use for the rest of your life. When you stop taking the medication, your cholesterol levels will return to premedication levels.

The NCEP has developed recommendations for lipid-lowering therapies that are primarily based on LDL-C concentrations (see table 7.1). Lipid-lowering medications combined with increased physical activity and a heart-healthy diet will optimize your blood total cholesterol, LDL-C, and HDL-C levels. Still, medications remain the core component for lowering blood lipids.

Table 7.1 LDL-C Goals for Drug Therapy

LDL goal	Initiation LDL level for lifestyle change	Drug therapy consideration
<100 mg/dL	>100 mg/dL	>130 mg/dL (100 to 129 mg/dL: drug optional)*
<130 mg/dL	>130 mg/dL	>130 mg/dL
<160 mg/dL	>160 mg/dL	>190 mg/dL (160 to 189 mg/dL: LDL-lowering drug optional)

*Some authorities recommend use of LDL-lowering medication in this category if an LDL-C <100 mg/dL cannot be achieved by lifestyle changes. Others prefer the use of drugs that primarily modify TG and HDL-C (nictonic acid or fibric acid).

From the National Heart, Lung and Blood Institute and the National Institutes of Health (NIH), a section of the US Department of Health and Human Services.

Lipid-Lowering Medications

For those individuals who are genetically predisposed to high blood cholesterol, are not able to lose weight, or have been unsuccessful in altering their diets or starting an exercise program, many drug therapies are available. These lipid-lowering medications include some that have been in use for many years as well as some relatively new drugs that are also very effective in controlling high blood cholesterol (see table 7.2).

Table 7.2 Lipid-Lowering Medications

Drug class	Generic name	Brand name
Blood cholesterol and LDL-C medications		
HMG-CoA reductase inhibitor	Atorvastatin	Lipitor
	Fluvastatin	Lescol
	Lovastatin	Mevacor
	Pravastatin	Pravachol
	Simvastatin	Zocor
	Rosuvastatin	Crestor
	Lovastatin + niacin	Advicor
Cholesterol-absorption inhibitors	Ezetimibe	Zetia
	Ezetimibe + simvastatin	Vytorin
Bile-acid sequestrants	Cholestyramine	Questran, Cholybar, Prevalite
	Colesevelam	Welchol
	Colestipol	Colestid
Nicotinic acid	Niacin	Niaspan, Nicobid, Slo-Niacin
Triglyceride-lowering medications		
Fibric acid derivatives	Clofibrate	Atromid
	Gemfibrozil	Lopid
	Fenofibrate	Tricor, Lofibra
Nicotinic acid	Niacin	Niaspan, Nicobid, Slo-Niacin

Adapted, by permission, from American College of Sports Medicine, 2005, *ACSM's guidelines for exercise testing and prescription*, 7th ed. (Baltimore, MD: Lippincott Williams & Wilkins), 258-259.

Cholesterol-lowering medications work in different ways. One class of drugs, 3-hydroxy-3-methylglutaryl coenzymeA reductase inhibitors (HMG CoA reductase inhibitors), or statins, affect blood cholesterol by reducing the amount of cholesterol made by the liver. Several other classes of drugs reduce the amount of cholesterol absorbed by the small intestine. For example, *bile-acid sequestrants* reduce the amount of cholesterol absorbed from intestinal bile acids. *Cholesterol-absorption inhibitors* (a new class of medications for cholesterol reduction) reduce the absorption of dietary cholesterol and fat. *Niacin,* a B-vitamin found in food and supplements, is used to treat high cholesterol by reducing the liver's production of cholesterol. Another class of lipid-lowering medications is *fibric acid derivatives,* which increase the action of an enzyme called lipoprotein lipase (which breaks down triglyceride-rich particles found in the walls of blood vessels of the cardiovascular system) and enhance cholesterol excretion as bile.

Side Effects of Lipid-Lowering Medications

Drug side effects are always a concern, but lipid-lowering medications in general are very safe. Still, it is important to understand the possible side effects of any drug you take. One potential side effect of lipid-lowering medications is liver injury or toxicity, but this is rarely a major problem. The liver is one of the few organs in the body that can repair itself when the injury is caught in the early stages. With careful monitoring of liver function through simple blood tests, it is rare for any cholesterol-lowering medication to cause an irreversible complication. Before you start any cholesterol-lowering drug, you should have a blood test for liver function. This test is usually repeated six weeks later and then every three to six months thereafter. Liver toxicity, which is often accompanied by nausea, fatigue, and abdominal discomfort, can typically be reversed by stopping the medication for several days. In some circumstances the medication can be restarted and continued at a lower dose. The best way to prevent or reduce side effects is to schedule regular follow-up visits with your doctor. These physician visits are important because they reduce the likelihood of long-term complications from the medications.

Another common side effect of lipid-lowering medications is muscle pain and discomfort that may be related to *rhabdomyolysis.* Rhabdomyolysis is a condition where muscle cells break down and release compounds such as myoglobin, a muscle protein, into the bloodstream. The kidneys filter myoglobin and the other compounds out of the body, but when large amounts of these compounds exist in the blood, the kidney is not able to process them. This inability to process the excess compounds ultimately leads to kidney failure, which leads to death. In very rare cases statin use has led to rhabdomyolysis and death (Hammer 2003).

Associated with rhabdomyolysis are elevations of a substance in the blood referred to as *creatine phosphokinase (CPK)*. This substance is released by tissues that are undergoing muscle protein breakdown. CPK is also released after strenuous exercise. When more exercise is completed, additional releases of CPK may occur with further increases in blood CPK, which may result in more muscle pain and discomfort. The problem is that sometimes lipid-lowering medications and exercise may both be causing muscle protein breakdown, and the only warning sign is constant muscle pain and discomfort. If you are taking a statin and have constant muscle pain, contact your doctor immediately. Even if you are exercising and you think the muscle pain is related to the exercise, contact your physician for follow-up tests.

Many heart disease patients undergo cardiac rehabilitation. A few patients undergoing cardiac rehabilitation may experience rhabdomyolysis with the use of statins. They may also be doing strenuous exercise and believe that the exercise is responsible for the muscle pain or discomfort, when the pain is more likely a result of rhabdomyolysis. Any unusual muscle pain or discomfort should be reported to your physician immediately. No other lipid-lowering medications have side effects with such direct implications for heart disease patients participating in exercise programs.

Rhabdomyolysis can also occur when a statin is used in combination with other agents such as fibric acid derivatives, niacin, cyclosporine, certain antibiotics, and fibric derivatives. Again, cholesterol-lowering medications, like any drugs, have side effects that can range from mild to serious depending on the individual. Some lipid-lowering medications can also adversely interact with other drugs. Hence, you should keep accurate and up-to-date records regarding all medications that you are taking and review this list each time you visit your physician.

Many lipid-lowering medications can cause muscle aches, abdominal pain, and constipation. Niacin can cause headaches and itchy skin. Bile-acid sequestrants have side effects similar to statins, namely upset stomach and constipation. A doctor can determine which medication is best for lowering your cholesterol while minimizing side effects.

Food and Exercise Interaction With Medications

Diet and exercise are the primary keys to healthy living. But in some cases, food and exercise interactions with medication can worsen the medication's side effects. For instance, grapefruit has often been praised for its ability to assist in weight loss, but it can interact with blood pressure medications to cause nausea, flushing of the face, dizziness, confusion, irregular heartbeat, and heart palpitations. At the same time grapefruit also can intensify the positive effects of medications, as is the case for statin medications. Eating grapefruit after taking a statin can cause the statin to have a greater lowering effect on cholesterol.

Exercise can have similar positive and negative effects as grapefruit. For example, aerobic exercise is thought to work positively with medications in controlling high blood pressure. On the other hand, patients taking statin medications to lower cholesterol complain of nonspecific muscle pain, tenderness, weakness, joint pains, and lupus-like symptoms, all of which are characteristic of rhabdomyolysis, a rare but serious problem that can occur with statin use (Hammer 2003), as discussed earlier. It is possible that high-intensity exercise interacts with statin medications to enhance the adverse rhabdomyolysis effects, which is a serious negative medication interaction.

Classes of Medications

Some cholesterol-lowering medications lower blood cholesterol and LDL-C levels while others lower only blood triglyceride levels. In general, most medications that lower blood cholesterol and LDL-C and triglycerides will also improve blood HDL-C (see table 7.3). In addition, several new cholesterol-lowering drugs are currently undergoing testing, and a number of well-tested lipid-lowering medications are now available in Europe. Eventually these medications will be available in the United States.

Another common practice used by physicians is prescribing several lipid-lowering drugs at once. This practice can cause substantial reductions in blood cholesterol and LDL-C levels and increases in HDL-C levels while reducing cost and side effects and enhancing compliance. However, some lipid-lowering medication combinations should be avoided. For example, statins and fibric acid derivatives should not be combined.

HMG-CoA Reductase Inhibitors

HMG-CoA reductase inhibitors, or statins, are usually selected as the initial lipid-lowering medication because they are extremely effective and work in most circumstances. Statins reduce the production of cholesterol by the liver, which causes an increase in the LDL receptors on most cells of the body. The combined effect is to decrease blood cholesterol and LDL-C. In addition, HMG-CoA reductase inhibitors have been shown to reduce first-time heart attacks as well as the likelihood of a second heart attack. Six statins are currently available in the United States: atorvastatin, cervistatin, fluvastatin, lovastatin, pravastatin, and simvastatin. More powerful statins with fewer side effects are under development and should be available for use in the next several years. Current statin drugs can reduce LDL-C by 20 to 60 percent while reducing blood triglycerides by as much as 40 percent and increasing HDL-C by 6 to 10 percent.

Table 7.3 Lipid-Lowering Medications and Their Mode of Action, Follow-Up, and Effect

Name	Mode of action	Follow-up	Effect
HMG-CoA reductase inhibitors	Particularly blocks liver enzyme HMG-CoA reductase, a cholesterol-production regulator.	Cholesterol profile and liver function tests checked at 6 and 12 weeks after and then every 6 months.	Reduction in total cholesterol and LDL-C levels, small reduction in TG, and slight increase in HDL-C.
Cholesterol-absorption inhibitors	Lipid-lowering compounds selectively inhibit the intestinal absorption of cholesterol and related phytosterols.	No liver function tests are required if used alone. When used in combination with a statin, follow statin recommendations.	Lowers TG, plasma cholesterol, and LDL-C with increases in HDL-C (more information is being collected).
Bile-acid sequestrants	Binds with bile acid (made from cholesterol) in the intestines to be excreted in stool.	No follow-up necessary.	Increases special LDL-removing receptors in liver cells. Lowers LDL-C by 15 to 30%.
Niacin	Lowers the liver's production of VLDL particles.	Blood tests to evaluate cholesterol response, liver function, blood sugar, and uric acid.	Lowers TG (30 to 40%) and LDL-C (15 to 30%), and increases HDL-C (15 to 25%).
Fibric acid	Increases lipoprotein lipase activity (breaks down triglyceride-rich particles) and amount of cholesterol excreted into bile. Appears to slow TG production in liver cells.	Tests for liver function and complete blood count within 6 weeks of starting the medication and 6 to 12 months thereafter.	Lowers TG by 25 to 60% and raises HDL-C by 15 to 25%.

Adapted, by permission, from S. Roach, 2005, *Pharmacology for health professionals* (Philadelphia, PA: Lippincott Williams & Wilkins), 244-254.

Statins have relatively few side effects. Some patients experience an upset stomach, flatulence, constipation, and abdominal pain or cramps. These symptoms usually are mild to moderate in severity and go away as your body adjusts to the statin. In a very few cases abnormalities show up in liver blood tests. Muscle aches and discomforts are also rare side effects. When symptoms like muscle soreness, pain, overall weakness or fatigue, or discolored urine occur, contact your doctor immediately for further blood tests.

Cholesterol-Absorption Inhibitors

The drug ezetimibe (Zetia) is the first in a new class of lipid-lowering agents referred to as cholesterol-absorption inhibitors. This class of drugs works to selectively inhibit cholesterol absorption from both intestinal bile acids and dietary sources in the small intestine. This reduced absorption decreases the delivery of intestinal cholesterol to the liver, which causes the liver to deplete its own cholesterol stores and increase the removal of cholesterol from the blood. This process for cholesterol removal complements the process that HMG-CoA reductase inhibitors use. Present information suggests that ezetimibe does not affect the absorption of fat-soluble vitamins like vitamins A and D and does not interfere with the production of steroid hormones. Reductions in blood cholesterol and LDL-C levels as a result of ezetimibe are approximately 15 to 25 percent.

Ezetimibe is FDA-approved for use with statins but not with other lipid-lowering medications. When used in combination with a statin, the production of cholesterol in the liver is blocked by reductions in the enzyme HMG-CoA reductase (because of the statin), and cholesterol absorption from the intestine. Few side effects have been reported, but the side effects that have been reported include stomach pain, diarrhea, fatigue, and in rare cases allergic reactions that require treatment right away, including swelling of the face, lips, tongue, and throat that may cause breathing and swallowing difficulties, rashes, muscle aches, alterations in some blood liver tests, and others. When ezetimibe is *not* used in conjunction with a statin, no follow-up liver tests are usually necessary. However, once ezetimibe and a statin are used together, follow-up guidelines for statin use should be followed.

Bile-Acid Sequestrants

Bile-acid sequestrant medications are prescribed in the form of a powdered resin in tablets or dissolved in liquid. The tablets often are not effective unless multiple tablets are taken. Bile-acid sequestrants inhibit the reabsorption of bile acid from the intestines and also reduce the transportation of bile acid to the liver. The loss of intestinal bile results in reduced blood cholesterol and LDL-C levels. Bile-acid sequestrants are most effective when taken with a fatty meal, because dietary fat increases bile production. The major side effects of bile-acid sequestrants are constipation, bloating, and flatulence. Bile-acid sequestrants also interfere with the absorption of fat-soluble vitamins and other medications. Newer forms of these drugs are being designed so that they do not interfere with the absorption of vitamins and other medications.

Bile-acid sequestrants are generally not prescribed as the sole medicine to lower cholesterol, especially if you have high triglycerides or a history of severe constipation. Although bile-acid sequestrants are not absorbed, they do interfere with the absorption of other medicines when taken at the same time. Other medications should be taken at least one hour before or four to six hours after the bile-acid resin. Talk with your doctor about the timing for taking bile-acid sequestrants when you're taking other medications as well. In addition, bile-acid sequestrant resins often increase blood triglyceride levels; however, this effect can be reduced by aerobic exercise.

Fibric Acid Derivatives

Fibric acid derivatives are useful for lowering elevated triglyceride levels. Gemfibrozil, clofibrate, and fenofibrate are currently available in the United States. Fibric acid derivatives can increase LDL-C levels slightly in patients who have very high triglyceride levels. The reason for this slight rise in LDL-C is that fibric acid increases lipoprotein lipase (LPL) activity, which facilitates the conversion of VLDL particles to LDL particles. Fibric acids should be used with extreme caution if you are taking a statin, because this combination can produce rhabdomyolysis. If you have a lipid disorder that warrants this type of drug combination, you should ask your doctor to help you find a lipid specialty clinic in order to properly manage your lipid disorder.

People using fibric acid generally report few side effects. When problems do occur, gastrointestinal complaints are the most common. Fibrates also appear to increase the likelihood of developing cholesterol gallstones. Fibrates can enhance the effect of medications like Coumadin (warfarin) that thin the blood.

Niacin or Nicotinic Acid

Niacin or nicotinic acid is extremely useful for patients with low HDL-C levels and is better than any of the other lipid-lowering agents in elevating blood HDL-C while also reducing LDL-C triglyceride levels. Another role of niacin is to limit the breakdown of lipids from fat cells, referred to as lipolysis. A reduction in lipolysis reduces free fatty acids in the blood, and reduced fatty acids limit the liver's ability to manufacture triglycerides. This reduction in blood fatty acid causes triglyceride levels to fall. Because lipolysis is greatest during periods of fasting such as overnight, the most important niacin dose is the bedtime dose. Sustained-release formulations of niacin designed solely for bedtime doses are available.

A common and troublesome side effect of nicotinic acid is flushing or hot flashes, which are the result of the niacin causing blood vessels to open wide. Most people adjust to the flushing in time, but for some the flushing can be decreased by taking the niacin during or after meals or taking aspirin or similar medications prescribed by your doctor. The extended or slow-release form of niacin usually causes less flushing than other forms of niacin.

If you are taking medications for high blood pressure, the action of these medicines may be enhanced by niacin and lower your blood pressure even more. You should monitor your blood pressure until you are used to your niacin regimen. Using the extended or slow-release form of niacin can minimize this condition.

A variety of gastrointestinal symptoms, including nausea, indigestion, flatulence, vomiting, diarrhea, and the activation of peptic ulcers, have been seen with the use of nicotinic acid. Three other major adverse effects include liver problems, gout, and high blood sugar. The risk of the latter three effects increases as the dose of nicotinic acid increases. Because of niacin's effect on blood sugar levels, your doctor may not prescribe this medicine to you if you have diabetes. All individuals treated with niacin should have liver function tests performed at least every four months, because niacin can produce reversible hepatitis, activate gout and peptic ulcers, and lead to *glucose intolerance.* Hepatitis is more frequent with sustained-release niacin, but it can occur with both forms of niacin. Patients should stop taking the medication and contact their physician if they develop frequent nausea or vomiting, unexpected weight loss, or other potential signs of hepatitis.

Non-Lipid-Lowering Medications

Some non-lipid-lowering medications used to treat other medical conditions can also affect blood lipid and lipoprotein levels. These other medications include beta antagonists (beta blockers), thiazine diuretics, oral hyperglycemic agents, insulin, estrogen, and progesterone. If you are taking these medications and your physician prescribes a lipid-lowering medication, discuss the potential for drug interactions with your physician.

Aspirin, a drug that has been used for centuries to relieve pain and reduce fever, has been shown to reduce the risk of future heart attacks in patients who have already had a heart attack. Aspirin works to reduce the risk of future heart attacks by reducing the stickiness of the platelets (the cells that cause blood clotting) so that blood clots do not form as readily. After bypass surgery, patients treated with aspirin have fewer early closures of the newly grafted blood vessels in the heart. Aspirin also reduces some of the side effects of niacin.

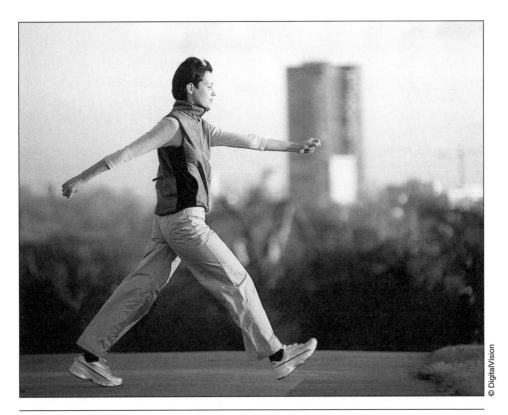

Be sure to talk to your doctor about possible interactions between your medication and exercise.

Beta blockers may increase blood triglyceride concentrations and reduce HDL-C levels except for those beta blockers containing intrinsic sympathomimetic actions. Thiazide is used as a diuretic and may increase total plasma cholesterol, VLDL-C, LDL-C, and triglycerides without affecting HDL-C concentration. Oral hypoglycemic agents or insulin therapy may reduce blood triglyceride levels and increase HDL-C levels in diabetic persons whose blood glucose is not controlled. These benefits are secondary to the improvement in blood glucose. Levothyroxine increases hepatic LDL receptor activity and thereby lowers blood LDL-C in people who have hypothyroidism. This medication may produce elevations of heart rate and blood pressure as well as cardiac dysrhythmias, and it can lead to angina in patients with heart disease. Oral contraceptives tend to increase blood cholesterol depending on the estrogen–progesterone ratio. Estrogen tends to increase blood HDL-C and VLDL triglyceride levels, especially in postmenopausal women, while progesterone decreases blood triglyceride and HDL-C levels.

Summary

Although therapeutic lifestyle interventions like exercise programming, a heart-healthy diet, and weight loss provide positive health benefits such as reduced blood cholesterol and LDL-C, the primary therapy for reducing blood cholesterol and LDL-C levels is medication. If you are diagnosed with high blood cholesterol, you should try these therapeutic lifestyle interventions before starting a lipid-lowering medication program. If you have not reached your blood lipid and lipoprotein goals after three to six months of these lifestyle interventions, you should then start a lipid-lowering medication program. When you start the medications, continue the exercise and heart-healthy diet programs, because they enhance the lipid-lowering medications' effects in addition to providing other health benefits.

Lipid-lowering medications are very effective and generally cause few side effects. Statin drugs are the first medication used in a lipid-lowering program, and drugs such as bile-acid sequestrants, fibric acid derivatives, and niacin are also effective. With new drugs in the developmental stages, people who require cholesterol-lowering medicines will soon have more choices and hopefully even greater success in normalizing cholesterol levels.

ACTION PLAN:

CHOOSING MEDICATION FOR LOWER CHOLESTEROL

- ☐ Develop your understanding of the use of lipid-lowering medications in reducing blood cholesterol and LDL-C.
- ☐ Gain knowledge concerning side effects of common lipid-lowering medications.
- ☐ Identify the different lipid-lowering medications and how they are used to reduce blood cholesterol and LDL-C.
- ☐ Learn about non-lipid-lowering medications.
- ☐ Ensure that you know of possible interactions among medications, diet, and exercise; if there are any questions, discuss them with your doctor.

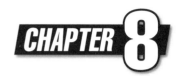

CHAPTER 8

INVESTIGATING COMPLEMENTARY AND ALTERNATIVE THERAPIES

In previous chapters we presented traditional methods for positively alter-ing blood cholesterol and LDL-C. However, some people are looking for ways outside these traditional methods to manage their blood cholesterol. Many approaches to health care exist that are not within the realm of con-ventional medicine as practiced in the United States. Currently, the National Center for Complementary and Alternative Medicine (NCCAM), a federal agency that is a component of the National Institutes of Health (NIH), is dedicated to bettering our understanding of complementary and alternative healing practices. This agency has developed a list of terms used to describe many of these medicines and practices (see the sidebar on pages 148-149). The NCCAM works to accomplish its stated objectives by encouraging rig-orous scientific investigation of nontraditional medicines and practices, encouraging the training of scientists in these areas, and making information available concerning complementary and alternative medicine.

Complementary medicine is used in conjunction with conventional medicine. An example of a complementary therapy is using fragrance treatment (aromatherapy) to help lessen a patient's discomfort after surgery. Alternative medicine is used instead of conventional medicine. An example of an alternative therapy is using a specific herb to treat

Text on pages 147 through 152 courtesy of the National Center for Complementary and Alternative Medicine, http://nccam.nih.gov/ (accessed 6/29/05).

high blood cholesterol instead of traditional lipid-lowering medications. Another term is integrative medicine, which refers to the combination of mainstream medical therapies and those alternative therapies for which there is high-quality scientific evidence of safety and effectiveness.

Complementary and alternative medicines (CAM) are a group of diverse medical and health care systems, practices, and products that are not currently considered part of traditional medicine. Despite the fact that there is some scientific evidence for some CAM therapies, many fundamental questions about these therapies are yet to be answered through well-designed scientific studies. Questions such as whether these therapies or practices are safe and whether they work for the medical conditions for which they are meant should be answered when you are considering the use of CAM therapies.

Terminology of Complementary and Alternative Medicine

Acupuncture is a method of healing developed in China beginning at least 2,000 years ago. Today, acupuncture describes a family of procedures involving stimulation of anatomical points on the body by a variety of techniques. American practices of acupuncture incorporate medical traditions from China, Japan, Korea, and other countries. The acupuncture technique that has been scientifically studied the most involves penetrating the skin with thin, solid, metallic needles that are manipulated by the hands or by electrical stimulation.

Aromatherapy involves the use of essential oils (extracts or essences) from flowers, herbs, and trees to promote health and well-being.

Ayurveda is an alternative medical system that has been practiced primarily in the Indian subcontinent for 5,000 years. Ayurveda includes diet and herbal remedies and emphasizes the use of body, mind, and spirit in disease prevention and treatment.

Chiropractic is an alternative medical system that focuses on the relationship between bodily structure (primarily the spine) and function and how that relationship affects the preservation and restoration of health. Chiropractors use manipulative therapy as an integral treatment tool.

Dietary supplements. Congress defined the term dietary supplement in the Dietary Supplement Health and Education Act (DSHEA) of 1994. A dietary supplement is a product (other than tobacco) taken by mouth that contains a "dietary ingredient" intended to supplement the diet. Dietary ingredients may include vitamins, minerals, herbs or other botanicals, and amino acids, as well as substances such as enzymes, organ tissues, and metabolites. Dietary supplements come in many forms, including extracts, concentrates, tablets, capsules, gel caps, liquids, and powders. They have special requirements for labeling. Under DSHEA, dietary supplements are considered foods, not drugs.

Electromagnetic fields (EMFs, also called electric and magnetic fields) are invisible lines of force that surround all electrical devices. The earth also produces EMFs—electric fields are produced in thunderstorm activity, and magnetic fields are believed to be produced by electric currents flowing at the Earth's core.

Homeopathy is an alternative medical system based on the belief that "like cures like," meaning that small, highly diluted quantities of medicinal substances are prescribed to cure symptoms when the same substances given at higher or more concentrated doses would actually cause those symptoms.

Massage involves the manipulation of muscle and connective tissue to enhance the functioning of those tissues and promote relaxation and well-being.

Naturopathy is an alternative medical system that proposes a healing power in the body that establishes, maintains, and restores health. Practitioners work with the patient to support this power through treatments such as nutrition and lifestyle counseling, dietary supplements, medicinal plants, exercise, homeopathy, and treatments from traditional Chinese medicine.

Osteopathic medicine is a form of conventional medicine that emphasizes diseases arising in the musculoskeletal system. There is an underlying belief that all of the body's systems work together and disturbances in one system may affect function elsewhere in the body. Some osteopathic physicians practice osteopathic manipulation, a full-body system of hands-on techniques to alleviate pain, restore function, and promote health and well-being.

Qi gong is a component of traditional Chinese medicine that combines movement, meditation, and regulation of breathing to enhance the flow of qi (vital energy, pronounced "chee") in the body, improve blood circulation, and enhance immune function.

Reiki is a Japanese word referring to universal life energy. Reiki is based on the belief that when spiritual energy is channeled through a Reiki practitioner, the patient's spirit is healed, which in turn heals the physical body.

Therapeutic touch is derived from an ancient technique called "laying on of hands." It is based on the premise that the healing force of the therapist affects the patient's recovery; healing is promoted when the body's energies are in balance; and by passing their hands over the patient, healers can identify energy imbalances.

Traditional Chinese medicine (TCM) is the current name for an ancient system of health care from China. TCM is based on a concept of balanced qi, or vital energy, that is believed to flow throughout the body. Qi is proposed to regulate a person's spiritual, emotional, mental, and physical balance and is influenced by the opposing forces of yin (negative energy) and yang (positive energy). Disease is thought to result from disruptions in the flow of qi and yin and yang becoming imbalanced. Among the components of TCM are herbal and nutritional therapy, restorative physical exercises, meditation, acupuncture, and remedial massage.

Categories for Complementary and Alternative Medicine

The NCCAM defines the key categories used in the field of complementary and alternative medicine. In this section we'll describe these five categories.

Alternative medical systems. Alternative medical systems are built upon complete systems of theory and practice. Often these systems have evolved apart from and earlier than the conventional medical approach used in the United States. Examples of alternative medical systems that have developed in Western cultures include homeopathic medicine and naturopathic medicine. Examples of systems that have developed in non-Western cultures include traditional Chinese medicine and ayurveda.

Mind–body interventions. Mind–body medicine uses a variety of techniques to enhance the mind's capacity to affect bodily function and symptoms. Some techniques that were considered to be CAM in the past have become mainstream, such as patient support groups and cognitive-behavioral therapy. Other mind–body techniques are still considered to be CAM, including meditation, prayer, mental healing, and therapies that use creative outlets such as art, music, or dance.

Biologically based therapies. Biologically based therapies use substances found in nature, such as herbs, foods, and vitamins. Some examples include dietary supplements, herbal products, and so-called natural but as yet scientifically unproven therapies (for example, using shark cartilage to treat cancer).

Manipulative and body-based methods. Manipulative and body-based methods are based on manipulation and movement of one or more parts of the body. Some examples include chiropractic or osteopathic manipulation and massage.

Energy therapies. Energy therapies involve the use of energy fields. They are of two types, biofield therapies and bioelectromagnetic-based therapies.

• Biofield therapies are intended to affect energy fields that surround and penetrate the human body. The existence of such fields has not yet been scientifically proven. Some forms of energy therapy manipulate biofields by applying pressure or manipulating the body by placing the hands in or through these fields. Examples include qi gong, Reiki, and therapeutic touch.

• Bioelectromagnetic-based therapies involve the unconventional use of electromagnetic fields, such as pulsed fields, magnetic fields, or alternating-current or direct-current fields.

Being Informed About Your Options

If you are considering using complementary or alternative medicine to treat your high blood cholesterol rather than the conventional medical means already discussed in this book, you should visit NCCAM's Web site (http://nccam.nih.gov/health/decisions/index.htm). This site was developed to aid you in your decision-making process about whether to use complementary and alternative medicines. See also the sidebar on page 152 on how to evaluate a Web site. Some key points you should consider when going through this decision-making process include the following:

• Regardless of whether you turn to a complementary or alternative medicine, you should take charge of your health by being an informed consumer. If you are going to be taking medication as discussed in chapter 7, you should find out what scientific studies have been done on the safety and effectiveness of the medication. In the same regard, you should determine what scientists have to say about the safety and effectiveness of the CAM therapy that you are considering.

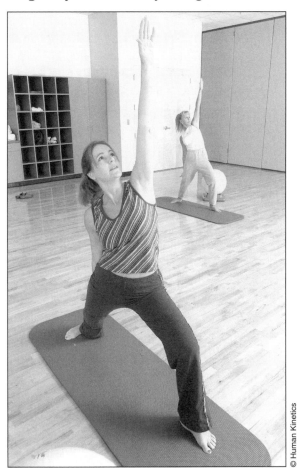

• In making decisions about your medical care and treatment, especially the use of CAM therapies, you should always consult with your health care provider to help you account for your individual needs.

• If you use any CAM therapy, always inform your primary health care provider right away. This is for your safety so that your

Meditative practices such as yoga are often used as CAMs to alleviate stress and other health problems.

health care provider can include the CAM therapy in your comprehensive treatment plan.

• If you use a CAM therapy provided by a practitioner, such as acupuncture, choose the practitioner with care. Check with your insurer to see if the services are reimbursable.

Evaluating a Web Site

Before following any medical advice from a Web site, you should make sure the information is accurate. Here are some questions to help you determine the credibility of a Web site:

• Who runs the site? Is it a government, university, or reputable medical or health-related association? Is it sponsored by a manufacturer of products or drugs? It should be easy to identify the sponsor of the site. If the site is government-run and sponsored, the credibility of the site is usually greater, and there is less likelihood of bias than if it's sponsored by a specific drug manufacturer. For example, if a drug company sponsors a Web site, the site may only recommend their own medications.

• What is the purpose of the site? Is it to educate the public or to sell a product? The purpose should be clearly stated. Again, sites run by drug manufacturers are often trying to sell their products and will usually give more favorable information that could be biased.

• What is the basis of the information? Is it based on scientific evidence with clear references? Advice and opinions should be clearly set apart from the science.

• How current is the information? Is it reviewed and updated frequently? Check out the listing of when the site was most recently updated. If none exists or the last update was several years old, this should cast doubt as to the site's accuracy and credibility.

For more tips on evaluating information on the Web, read NCCAM's "10 Things to Know About Evaluating Medical Resources on the Web," which can be found at http://nccam.nih.gov/health/webresources/.

Choosing a Lipid-Lowering Complementary or Alternative Medicine

Physicians and allied health practitioners are giving greater consideration to complementary and alternative therapies in their attempt to develop a comprehensive approach to health care that is as effective as medication but without the side effects. As with any traditional therapy, the overall goal of a CAM therapy is to use nonconventional approaches that will lead to a better quality of life and well-being.

Complementary or alternative methods and products to lower blood cholesterol and LDL-C include herbal products and nutritional supplements. Some of these products have scientific data that are reliable and are consistent in showing a substantial health benefit, while others have contradictory, insufficient, or preliminary information that at best only suggests a health benefit. In some cases herbal products and nutritional supplements are supported only by traditional recommendations with little or no scientific data available supporting their use.

For many people, the use of herbal products and nutritional supplements is complicated by conflicting claims of effectiveness and safety, political and economic interests, a lack of scientific investigation, the absence of federal regulation, a lack of quality control during production, and most of all, a lack of reliable sources of valid consumer information. Because the FDA does not regulate herbal compounds as it regulates drugs in the United States, these substances may be sold as food additives. A major concern is that companies selling these products claim effectiveness for treating specific medical conditions without the necessary supportive research data. Before taking any herbal product or supplement, you should use all means available to find as much information as possible about the product. At the very least, this includes reading product labels, if they are included. However, product labels may be misleading, or they may simply express the health purpose of the product or some other nonspecific purpose. Frequently, there are few directions on how to use the product or what precautions to take. Because there is a lack of customer information, consumers must place their trust solely in the manufacturer's advertisement. However, some nutritional supplement manufacturers voluntarily comply with the FDA's Good Manufacturing Practices required of pharmaceutical companies, while many other manufacturers do not.

Herbal Products As Lipid-Lowering Agents

Herbal products are not drugs, and from a regulatory and legal viewpoint, in the United States these compounds are basically self-prescribed and therefore do not come under federal regulatory control. Herbal compounds have been used as traditional medicines for centuries by tribal healing practitioners in many cultures, and in some countries, these herbal products are prescribed by licensed physicians for specific purposes. Herbal products also may have positive health effects for some users but not necessarily all users. Herbal products can have serious side effects, particularly if used in combination with prescribed medications for the same medical condition or an unrelated condition (for an example, see the sidebar on page 155 on grapefruit, grapefruit juice, and Seville oranges).

We will discuss some of the herbal products used to treat elevated blood cholesterol and LDL-C, but many more products are available than what we will discuss. By presenting this list, we do not imply endorsement for use, safety, or effectiveness. Rather, we present this list as a source for you as you begin to investigate complementary and alternative medicine for lowering blood cholesterol and LDL-C.

Red Yeast Rice

Red yeast rice is fermented by the red yeast *Monascus purpureus* and has been used by Chinese people for many centuries as a food preservative and colorant and as an ingredient in rice wine. In addition, red yeast rice has been used for more than 1,000 years as a medicine and more recently as an herbal product to lower blood cholesterol and triglyceride levels. Three different red yeast rice preparations are Zhitai, Cholestin, and Xuezhikang. All of these preparations contain a natural cholesterol-lowering substance that inhibits HMG-CoA reductase, an enzyme important for cholesterol production by the liver. Red yeast rice is very much like the statins that were discussed in chapter 7.

- Zhitai is produced by the fermentation of a mixture of *Monascus purpureaus* strains from whole-grain rice.
- Cholestin or HypoCol is produced by the fermentation of selected strains of *Monascus purpureaus* to produce monacolin K (monacolin K is a statin called lovastatin, which is a major cholesterol-lowering drug—see chapter 7).
- Xuezhikang is produced by mixing rice and red yeast with alcohol and processing the mixture to remove most of the rice gluten. Xuezhikang contains 40 percent more cholesterol-lowering ingredients than Cholestin.

Red yeast rice is effective in lowering blood cholesterol in people with elevated blood cholesterol levels. Zhitai and Xuezhikang are consistently associated with lower blood cholesterol by an average of 10 to 30 percent, lower LDL-C by an average of 10 to 20 percent, lower triglycerides by an average of 15 to 25 percent, and increased HDL by an average of 7 to 15 percent. Cholestin has been shown to reduce blood cholesterol, LDL-C, and triglyceride levels, but appears to have no effect on HDL-C. No damage was reported for the kidneys, liver, or other organs, and only rare and minor side affects such as heartburn or indigestion were reported with the use of red yeast rice (Heber et al. 1999). A limitation of these scientific trials is that the studies generally lasted only a few weeks or months. Thus, conclusive proof of long-term safety (over a period of many years of use) will have to wait until additional trials over longer periods of time are completed. On the other hand, scientists generally believe that red yeast rice is safe in the long-term since it has been used as a food for thousands of years in Asian countries without reports of problems.

Grapefruit, Grapefruit Juice, and Seville Oranges

When grapefruit or grapefruit juice is consumed along with statins or HMG-CoA reductase inhibitors, they enhance the effects of the medications and significantly increase blood levels of the drugs, leading to a greater chance of side effects and liver damage. Because red yeast rice appears to act in much the same way as these cholesterol-lowering drugs, you should avoid drinking grapefruit juice or eating grapefruit or grapefruit products such as marmalade while taking red yeast rice. Grapefruit, grapefruit juice, and Seville oranges (found in marmalades and other condiments but not in juice) may increase blood levels of statins and therefore increase the risk of side effects, including potential damage to the liver or muscle tissue.

Fenugreek

Fenugreek (*Trigonella foenum-graecum*) is a herb native to southern Europe and Asia and is one of the oldest cultivated plants used for medicine. It is widely grown today in Mediterranean countries, Argentina, France, India, North Africa, and the United States and is used as a food and condiment as well as a medicine. In recent years there is growing commercial interest in fenugreek as a lipid-lowering product. Fenugreek contains a steroid component and a pasty fiber that are thought to account for many of the beneficial effects of fenugreek. The steroid element likely inhibits intestinal absorption of cholesterol as well as liver cholesterol synthesis, while the pasty fiber may help lower blood sugar levels. As a result, lower blood cholesterol and blood sugar levels are found in people with moderate atherosclerosis and type 2 diabetes. Similar results were also found in a controlled clinical trial of patients with type 1 diabetes who have elevated blood cholesterol (Sharma et al. 1990). Fenugreek use did not affect blood HDL-C levels.

Psyllium

Psyllium or psyllium husks come from the crushed seeds of the *Plantago ovata* plant, an herb native to parts of Asia, Mediterranean regions of Europe, and North Africa. Psyllium seed husks are used in the preparation of many herbal remedies. Similar to oats and wheat, psyllium is rich in soluble fiber, so eating a small serving each day contributes the soluble fiber necessary to achieve a cholesterol-lowering effect. Psyllium is also a common ingredient in over-the-counter bulk laxative products. Numerous studies have found that psyllium supplementation can lower blood cholesterol and LDL-C levels while HDL-C levels remain unaffected. The cholesterol-lowering effect of psyllium has been reported in children as well as adults.

Artichoke

Artichoke is a large, thistle-like plant *(Cynara scolymus)* that is native to southern Europe, North Africa, and the Canary Islands. Artichoke leaves contain a number of active elements that are effective in treating mild indigestion. Artichoke extract consumed three times a day has been found to reduce nausea, abdominal pain, constipation, and flatulence. Artichoke extract is also used to treat high blood cholesterol and triglyceride levels. Scientists are not certain how artichoke leaves lower cholesterol, but reductions are thought to be caused by inhibition of cholesterol synthesis by the liver and reduced absorption of cholesterol from the intestine. Artichoke extract also prevents LDL-C oxidation, which can reduce the risk of heart disease.

Garlic

Garlic *(Allium sativum)* has been used as a medicine for centuries. Some research suggests that garlic may reduce blood cholesterol and triglyceride levels. However, the latest scientific literature supports only a small overall lipid-lowering effect. If you do decide to take garlic as a supplement, you can take specific preparation strategies to maximize its effect. One word of caution: Be careful in using garlic supplements. Consuming large amounts of garlic in food is unlikely to be harmful, but taking too much garlic in the form of supplements can lead to symptoms such as dizziness and fainting. Likewise, garlic supplements may not be a wise choice for everyone because of its anti-blood-clotting properties. If you take anticoagulant (blood-thinner) drugs, you should check with your doctor before taking garlic supplements, and if you are considering any type of surgery, you should inform your surgeon that you are taking garlic supplements. Finally, certain medicines may interact with garlic. Before taking any new medicines, you should inform your doctor that you are taking garlic supplements.

Green Tea

Green, black, and oolong (shares qualities of both green and black) teas are derived from the same plant, *Camellia sinensis,* but the difference between green tea and other teas is in how the leaves are processed and prepared. Green tea is not fermented; black and oolong teas are. As a result, the active ingredients in the herb remain unchanged. Many studies have found that green tea can slightly lower blood cholesterol levels and improve the lipoprotein cholesterol profile (decreases LDL-C while increasing HDL-C). However, not all scientific studies have confirmed this. Green tea has also been shown to protect against damage to LDL-C caused by oxidation. When LDL-C is oxidative, arterial wall LDL-C and plaque buildup are promoted. Consumption of green tea also increases blood antioxidant activity.

Guggul

The stem of the mukul myrrh tree *(Commiphora mukul)* yields a yellow-ish resin known as guggul and gum guggulu. The resin contains steroid compounds known as guggulsterones that provide cholesterol- and triglyceride-lowering actions. These actions render guggul as a significant agent in lowering blood triglyceride and cholesterol as well as LDL-C and VLDL-C levels while causing HDL-C levels to rise. Guggulsterones also are antioxidants that prevent LDL-C oxidation, thus protecting against heart disease. Guggul extract is similar to the drug clofibrate, which is also used for lowering blood cholesterol and LDL-C levels (see chapter 7).

Nutritional Supplements As Lipid-Lowering Agents

Nutritional supplements include any substance consumed to promote health or wellness. The FDA and Federal Trade Commission enforce current legislation prohibiting manufacturers from making specific claims of treating or curing disease without scientific proof, because some manufacturers may make untrue or unsubstantiated claims in order to boost sales.

The following discussion presents nutritional supplements that play an important role in lowering cholesterol and LDL-C and are not generally considered vitamins, minerals, or specific herbs. Nonetheless, each may contain some of the necessary nutrients to cause a reduction in blood cholesterol and LDL-C.

Beta-Glucan

Beta-glucan is found in the cell walls of baker's yeast, oat, wheat, barley fiber, cereals (bran), and some mushrooms. It's a complex sugar and a source of soluble fiber. Oat bran has been found to have a significant cholesterol-lowering effect, and beta-glucan is the key reason for this action. Because it's a soluble fiber, beta-glucan binds cholesterol and bile acids and assists in the elimination of these molecules from the body, which effectively helps reduce blood cholesterol. Scientific studies evaluating use of either oat- or yeast-derived beta-glucan for at least four weeks found reductions of approximately 10 percent in blood cholesterol and 8 percent in LDL-C and elevations in HDL-C ranging from 0 to 16 percent (Nicolosi et al. 1999; Behall et al. 1997).

Vitamin Supplements

Beta-carotene (vitamin A), vitamin C, vitamin E, and selenium are antioxidants that help to protect the heart in two ways. First, these vitamins enter the LDL-C molecules and block the harmful chemical process of oxidation. With oxidation blocked, cholesterol is less likely to contribute to plaque buildup in the arteries. Second, antioxidants can block the effects of oxygen-free radicals. Oxygen-free radicals are present as either the by-products of metabolism or as substances from air pollution or tobacco smoke. Radicals are harmful to the heart because they are thought to promote the buildup of plaque in arteries. When the development of free radicals is blocked, the risk of heart disease is reduced. Because antioxidants have shown these heart-friendly effects, some researchers hail them as invaluable in the fight against heart disease. But some scientific research has shown only minimal or no effects from antioxidants. Much work currently is under way in the study of antioxidants' ability to reduce the risk of heart disease.

Three B-vitamins (vitamin B_6, vitamin B_{12}, and folic acid) have been identified as possible aids in reducing the risk of heart disease and stroke. These B-vitamins reduce homocysteine in the blood. Homocysteine, an amino acid, is a product of normal cellular processes, but too much homocysteine in the blood reflects an abnormal condition that can lead to increased risk of heart disease. A heart-healthy diet that includes at least five servings of fruits and vegetables a day contains enough vitamin B_6, vitamin B_{12}, and folic acid to reduce blood homocysteine levels and risk of heart disease. Citrus fruits, tomatoes, vegetables, and grain products are good sources of vitamin B_6, vitamin B_{12}, and folic acid.

Vitamin B_3, also known as niacin, is an accepted medical treatment for elevated cholesterol. The best food sources of vitamin B_3 are peanuts, brewer's yeast, fish, meat, and whole grains. Slow- or extended-release forms of niacin are preferable since they reduce the side effect of skin flushing. Niacin as a lipid-lowering prescription medication was discussed in chapter 7, but niacin is also available over the counter.

Coenzyme Q10

Coenzyme Q10 (CoQ10) is a naturally occurring nutrient found in all body cells and is obtained from almost all foods, particularly fish and other meats. Many people who take CoQ10 find that they are less likely to be fatigued, because CoQ10 plays a significant role in the cell's energy system. CoQ10 also has a role in improving certain types of cardiovascular diseases, including congestive heart failure and hypertension. Blood cholesterol levels are lower in some people taking coenzyme Q10, and it has also been shown to be an excellent antioxidant, preventing LDL-C from being oxidized.

CoQ10 levels in the blood are lowered in people taking statin drugs. As discussed in chapter 7, the statin drugs (e.g., lovastatin, pravastatin, and simvastatin) are prescription medications used to treat high blood cholesterol and LDL-C levels. These medications work by inhibiting an enzyme known as HMG-CoA reductase and are very effective in lowering cholesterol levels. However, HMG-CoA reductase is also responsible for the production of both coenzyme A (CoA) and coenzyme Q10. As a result, the cholesterol-lowering effect of these drugs is accompanied by a lowering of CoA and CoQ10 levels in both the cell and the blood. CoA and CoQ10 supplements may help to prevent some of the adverse effects of these widely used statins, and if you are taking a statin or red yeast rice you should consider taking CoQ10 supplements.

Summary

Several complementary and alternative therapies exist for lowering blood cholesterol and LDL-C levels. As with any lipid-lowering intervention, the primary goal of a CAM therapy is to lower your blood cholesterol and LDL-C and reduce your risk for heart disease, leading to a better quality of life. Though many of these complementary and alternative approaches are effective at lowering blood cholesterol without the side effects of some prescribed lipid-lowering medications, you should always consult your doctor about the particular approach that you plan to use. You and your doctor can devise a comprehensive approach to meet your specific needs and reduce the likelihood of any side effects. Many CAM therapies have not undergone the rigorous scientific study that traditional methods have experienced. Use as many different sources as possible in gathering available information regarding the different CAM therapies for lowering blood cholesterol and LDL-C.

In previous chapters you learned about the different therapeutic lifestyle interventions, including exercise programming, a heart-healthy diet, and weight loss, in providing positive health benefits to reduce your blood cholesterol and LDL-C levels. As discussed in earlier chapters, if after three to six months of these lifestyle interventions you have not reached your blood lipid LDL-C goals, you should then start a lipid-lowering medication program with the supervision of your physician. When using lipid-lowering medications, you should continue to exercise, eat a heart-healthy diet, and proceed with your CAM therapy, because these lifestyle programs will likely enhance the effects of lipid-lowering medications as well as provide other important health benefits.

ACTION PLAN:
INVESTIGATING COMPLEMENTARY AND ALTERNATIVE

☐ Learn the five categories of complementary and alternative medicines, and the terminology associated with these therapies.

☐ Follow guidelines for obtaining accurate and reliable information about different medicines, especially when seeking information from Web sites.

☐ Investigate herbal products as a means of lowering cholesterol; be sure to research each product carefully and be aware of negative side effects.

☐ Look into supplements for lowering cholesterol, but as with herbal products, be careful in your choice and do as much research as possible.

APPENDIX: LOW-CHOLESTEROL RECIPES

Bean and Macaroni Soup

2 16-oz. cans great northern beans

1 Tbsp. olive oil

1/2 lb. fresh mushrooms, sliced

1 c. onion, coarsely chopped

2 c. carrots, sliced

1 c. celery, coarsely chopped

1 clove garlic, minced

3 c. tomatoes, fresh, peeled, cut up (or 1 1/2 lb. canned, cut up)*

1 tsp. dried sage

1 tsp. dried thyme

1/2 tsp. dried oregano

black pepper, freshly ground, to taste

1 bay leaf, crumbled

4 c. elbow macaroni, cooked

*If using canned tomatoes, sodium content will be higher. Try no salt added canned tomatoes to keep sodium lower.

Drain beans and reserve liquid. Rinse beans. Heat oil in 6-quart kettle. Add mushrooms, onion, carrots, celery, and garlic and sauté for 5 minutes. Add tomatoes, sage, thyme, oregano, pepper, and bay leaf. Cover and cook over medium heat for 20 minutes.

Cook macaroni according to package directions, using unsalted water. Drain when cooked. Do not overcook.

Combine reserved bean liquid with water to make 4 cups. Add liquid, beans, and cooked macaroni to vegetable mixture. Bring to boil. Cover and simmer until soup is thoroughly heated. Stir occasionally.

Yield: 16 servings; serving size: 1 cup

Each serving provides: Calories: 158; total fat: 1 g; saturated fat: less than 1 g; cholesterol: 0 mg; sodium: 154 mg; total fiber: 5 g; protein: 8 g; carbohydrate: 29 g; potassium: 524 mg

All recipes taken from *Keep the Beat: Heart Healthy Recipes*, courtesy of the NHLBI (National Heart, Lung, and Blood Institute).

Corn Chowder

1 Tbsp. vegetable oil

2 Tbsp. celery, finely diced

2 Tbsp. onion, finely diced

2 Tbsp. green pepper, finely diced

1 10-oz. package frozen whole kernel corn

1 c. raw potatoes, peeled, diced into 1/2-inch pieces

2 Tbsp. fresh parsley, chopped

1 c. water

1/4 tsp. salt

black pepper, to taste

1/4 tsp. paprika

2 Tbsp. flour

2 c. low-fat or skim milk

Heat oil in medium saucepan. Add celery, onion, and green pepper, and sauté for 2 minutes. Add corn, potatoes, water, salt, pepper, and paprika. Bring to boil, then reduce heat to medium. Cook covered for about 10 minutes or until potatoes are tender.

Place 1/2 cup of milk in jar with tight-fitting lid. Add flour and shake vigorously. Gradually add milk-flour mixture to cooked vegetables. Then add remaining milk.

Cook, stirring constantly, until mixture comes to a boil and thickens. Serve garnished with chopped parsley.

Yield: 4 servings; serving size: 1 cup

Each serving provides: Calories: 186; total fat: 5 g; saturated fat: 1 g; cholesterol: 5 mg; sodium: 205 mg; total fiber: 4 g; protein: 7 g; carbohydrate: 31 g; potassium: 455 mg

Meatball Soup

1/2 lb. ground chicken

1/2 lb. lean ground beef

10 c. water

1 bay leaf

1 small onion, chopped

1/2 c. green pepper, chopped

1 tsp. mint

2 small tomatoes, chopped

1/2 tsp. oregano

4 Tbsp. instant corn flour

1/2 tsp. black pepper

2 cloves garlic, minced

1/2 tsp. salt

2 medium carrots, chopped

2 c. cabbage, chopped

2 celery stalks, chopped

1 10-oz. package frozen corn

2 medium zucchini, chopped

1 medium chayote, chopped (extra zucchini can be used instead)

1/2 c. cilantro, minced

In large pot, combine water, bay leaf, half of onion, green pepper, and 1/2 teaspoon of mint. Bring to boil.

In bowl, combine chicken, beef, other half of onion, tomato, oregano, corn flour, pepper, garlic, and salt. Mix well. Form 1-inch meatballs. Place meatballs in boiling water and lower heat. Cook over low heat for 30 to 45 minutes.

Add carrots, chayote, cabbage, and celery. Cook over low heat for 25 minutes. Add corn and zucchini. Cook for another 5 minutes. Garnish with cilantro and rest of mint.

Yield: 8 servings; serving size: 1 1/4 cups

Each serving provides: Calories: 161; total fat: 4 g; saturated fat: 1 g; cholesterol: 31 mg; sodium: 193 mg; total fiber: 4 g; protein: 13 g; carbohydrate: 17 g; potassium: 461 mg

Quick Beef Casserole

1/2 lb. lean ground beef

1 c. onion, chopped

1 c. celery, chopped

1 c. green pepper, cubed

3 1/2 c. tomatoes, diced

1/4 tsp. salt

1/2 tsp. black pepper

1/4 tsp. paprika

1 c. frozen peas

2 small carrots, diced

1 c. uncooked rice

1 1/2 c. water

In skillet, brown ground beef and drain off fat. Add rest of ingredients. Mix well. Cover and cook over medium heat until boiling. Reduce to low heat and simmer for 35 minutes. Serve hot.

Yield: 8 servings; serving size: 1 1/3 cups

Each serving provides: Calories: 201; total fat: 5 g; saturated fat: 2 g; cholesterol: 16 mg; sodium: 164 mg; total fiber: 3 g; protein: 9 g; carbohydrate: 31 g; potassium: 449 mg

Stir-Fried Beef and Chinese Vegetables

2 Tbsp. dry red wine

1 Tbsp. soy sauce

1/2 tsp. sugar

1 1/2 tsp. gingerroot, peeled, grated

1 lb. boneless round steak, fat trimmed, cut across grain into
    1 1/2-inch strips

2 Tbsp. vegetable oil

2 medium onions, cut into 8 wedges each

1/2 lb. fresh mushrooms, rinsed, trimmed, sliced

2 stalks (1/2 c.) celery, bias cut into 1/4-inch slices

2 small green peppers, cut into thin lengthwise strips

1 c. water chestnuts, drained, sliced

2 Tbsp. cornstarch

1/4 c. water

Prepare marinade by mixing together wine, soy sauce, sugar, and ginger. Marinate meat in mixture while preparing vegetables.

Heat 1 tablespoon oil in large skillet or wok. Stir-fry onions and mushrooms for 3 minutes over medium-high heat. Add celery and cook for 1 minute. Add remaining vegetables and cook for 2 minutes or until green pepper is tender but crisp. Transfer vegetables to warm bowl.

Add remaining 1 tablespoon oil to skillet. Stir-fry meat in oil for about 2 minutes, or until meat loses its pink color.

Blend cornstarch and water. Stir into meat. Cook and stir until thickened. Then return vegetables to skillet. Stir gently and serve.

Yield: 6 servings; serving size: 6 oz.

Each serving provides: Calories: 200; total fat: 9 g; saturated fat: 2 g; cholesterol: 40 mg; sodium: 201 mg; total fiber: 3 g; protein: 17 g; carbohydrate: 12 g; potassium: 552 mg

Chicken and Rice

6 chicken pieces (legs and breasts), skinless

2 tsp. vegetable oil

4 c. water

2 tomatoes, chopped

1/2 c. green pepper, chopped

1/4 c. red pepper, chopped

1/4 c. celery, diced

1 medium carrot, grated

1/4 c. frozen corn

1/2 c. onion, chopped

1/4 c. fresh cilantro, chopped

2 cloves garlic, finely chopped

1/8 tsp. salt

1/8 tsp. pepper

2 c. rice

1/2 c. frozen peas

2 oz. Spanish olives

1/4 c. raisins

In large pot, brown chicken pieces in oil. Add water, tomatoes, green and red peppers, celery, carrots, corn, onion, cilantro, garlic, salt, and pepper. Cover and cook over medium heat for 20 to 30 minutes or until chicken is done.

Remove chicken from pot and place in refrigerator. Add rice, peas, and olives to pot. Cover pot and cook over low heat for about 20 minutes until rice is done. Add chicken and raisins, and cook for another 8 minutes.

Yield: 6 servings; serving size: 1 cup of rice and 1 piece of chicken

Each serving provides: Calories: 448; total fat: 7 g; saturated fat: 2 g; cholesterol: 49 mg; sodium: 352 mg; total fiber: 4 g; protein: 24 g; carbohydrate: 70 g; potassium: 551 mg

Spaghetti With Turkey Meat Sauce

1 lb. lean ground turkey

1 28-oz. can tomatoes, cut up

1 c. green pepper, finely chopped

1 c. onion, finely chopped

2 cloves garlic, minced

1 tsp. dried oregano, crushed

1 tsp. black pepper

1 lb. spaghetti, uncooked

nonstick cooking spray

Coat large skillet with nonstick spray. Preheat over high heat. Add turkey and cook, stirring occasionally, for 5 minutes. Drain and discard fat. Stir in tomatoes with juice, green pepper, onion, garlic, oregano, and black pepper. Bring to boil. Reduce heat and simmer covered for 15 minutes, stirring occasionally. Remove cover and simmer for added 15 minutes. (For creamier sauce, give sauce a whirl in blender or food processor.)

Meanwhile, cook spaghetti in unsalted water. Drain well. Serve sauce over spaghetti.

Yield: 6 servings; serving size: 5 oz. of sauce with 9 oz. of cooked spaghetti

Each serving provides: Calories: 455; total fat: 6 g; saturated fat: 1 g; cholesterol: 51 mg; sodium: 248 mg; total fiber: 5 g; protein: 28 g; carbohydrate: 71 g; potassium: 593 mg

Mediterranean Baked Fish

1 lb. fish fillets (sole, flounder, or sea perch)

2 tsp. olive oil

1 large onion, sliced

1 16-oz. can whole tomatoes, drained (reserve juice), coarsely chopped

1/2 c. tomato juice (reserved from canned tomatoes)

1 bay leaf

1 clove garlic, minced

1 c. dry white wine

1/4 c. lemon juice

1/4 c. orange juice

1 Tbsp. fresh orange peel, grated

1 tsp. fennel seeds, crushed

1/2 tsp. dried oregano, crushed

1/2 tsp. dried thyme, crushed

1/2 tsp. dried basil, crushed

black pepper, to taste

Heat oil in large nonstick skillet. Add onion and sauté over medium heat for 5 minutes or until soft. Add all remaining ingredients except fish. Stir well and simmer uncovered for 30 minutes.

Arrange fish in 10- by 6-inch baking dish. Cover with sauce. Bake uncovered at 375° F for about 15 minutes or until fish flakes easily.

Yield: 4 servings; serving size: 4-oz. fillet with sauce

Each serving provides: Calories: 178; total fat: 4 g; saturated fat: 1 g; cholesterol: 56 mg; sodium: 260 mg; total fiber: 3 g; protein: 22 g; carbohydrate: 12 g; potassium: 678 mg

Scallop Kabobs

3 medium green peppers, cut into 1 1/2-inch squares

1 1/2 lb. fresh bay scallops

1 pt. cherry tomatoes

1/4 c. dry white wine

1/4 c. vegetable oil

3 Tbsp. lemon juice

dash garlic powder

black pepper, to taste

4 skewers

Parboil green peppers for 2 minutes. Alternately thread first three ingredients onto skewers. Combine next five ingredients. Brush kabobs with wine/oil/lemon mixture, then place on grill (or under broiler). Grill for 15 minutes, turning and basting frequently.

Yield: 4 servings; serving size: 1 kabob (6 oz.)

Each serving provides: Calories: 224; total fat: 6 g; saturated fat: 1 g; cholesterol: 43 mg; sodium: 355 mg; total fiber: 3 g; protein: 30 g; carbohydrate: 13 g; potassium: 993 mg

Tuna Salad

2 6-oz. cans tuna, water pack

1/2 c. celery, chopped

1/3 c. green onions, chopped

6 1/2 Tbsp. mayonnaise, reduced fat

Rinse and drain tuna for 5 minutes. Break apart with fork. Add celery, onion, and mayonnaise, and mix well.

Yield: 5 servings; serving size: 1/2 cup

Each serving provides: Calories: 146; total fat: 7 g; saturated fat: 1 g; cholesterol: 25 mg; sodium: 158 mg; total fiber: 1 g; protein: 16 g; carbohydrate: 4 g; potassium: 201 mg

Sweet and Sour Seashells

1 lb. uncooked small seashell pasta

2 Tbsp. vegetable oil

3/4 c. sugar

1/2 c. cider vinegar

1/2 c. wine vinegar

1/2 c. water

3 Tbsp. prepared mustard

black pepper, to taste

1 2-oz. jar sliced pimentos

2 small cucumbers

2 small onions, thinly sliced

18 leaves of lettuce

Cook pasta in unsalted water, drain, rinse with cold water, and drain again. Stir in oil. Transfer to 4-quart bowl.

In blender, place sugar, vinegars, water, prepared mustard, salt, pepper, and pimento. Process at low speed for 15 to 20 seconds, or just enough so flecks of pimento can be seen. Pour over pasta.

Score cucumber peel with fork tines. Cut cucumber in half lengthwise, then slice thinly. Add to pasta with onion slices. Toss well.

Marinate, covered, in refrigerator for 24 hours. Stir occasionally. Drain, and serve on lettuce.

Yield: 18 servings; serving size: 1/2 cup

Each serving provides: Calories: 158; total fat: 2 g; saturated fat: less than 1 g; cholesterol: 0 mg; sodium: 35 mg; total fiber: 2 g; protein: 4 g; carbohydrate: 31 g; potassium: 150 mg

Black Beans With Rice

1 lb. black beans, dry

7 c. water

1 medium green pepper, coarsely chopped

1 1/2 c. onion, chopped

1 Tbsp. vegetable oil

2 bay leaves

1 clove garlic, minced

1/2 tsp. salt

1 Tbsp. vinegar (or lemon juice)

6 c. rice, cooked in unsalted water

1 4-oz. jar sliced pimento, drained

1 lemon, cut into wedges

Pick through beans to remove bad ones. Soak beans overnight in cold water. Drain and rinse. In large soup pot or Dutch oven, stir together beans, water, green pepper, onion, oil, bay leaves, garlic, and salt. Cover and boil for 1 hour.

Reduce heat and simmer, covered, for 3 to 4 hours or until beans are very tender. Stir occasionally, and add water if needed. Remove and mash about a third of beans. Return to pot. Stir and heat through.

When ready to serve, remove bay leaves and stir in vinegar or lemon juice. Serve over rice. Garnish with sliced pimento and lemon wedges.

Yield: 6 servings; serving size: 8 oz.

Each serving provides: Calories: 508; total fat: 4 g; saturated fat: 1 g; cholesterol: 0 mg; sodium: 206 mg; total fiber: 14 g; protein: 21 g; carbohydrate: 98 g; potassium: 852 mg

Summer Vegetable Spaghetti

2 c. small yellow onions, cut in eighths

2 c. (about 1 lb.) ripe tomatoes, peeled, chopped

2 c. (about 1 lb.) yellow and green squash, thinly sliced

1 1/2 c. (about 1/2 lb.) fresh green beans, cut

2/3 c. water

2 Tbsp. fresh parsley, minced

1 clove garlic, minced

1/2 tsp. chili powder

1/4 tsp. salt

black pepper, to taste

1 6-oz. can tomato paste

1 lb. spaghetti, uncooked

1/2 c. Parmesan cheese, grated

Combine first 10 ingredients in large saucepan. Cook for 10 minutes, then stir in tomato paste. Cover and cook gently for 15 minutes, stirring occasionally, until vegetables are tender.

Cook spaghetti in unsalted water, according to package directions. Spoon sauce over drained hot spaghetti. Sprinkle Parmesan cheese on top.

Yield: 9 servings; serving size: 1 cup of spaghetti and 3/4 cup of sauce with vegetables

Each serving provides: Calories: 271; total fat: 3 g; saturated fat: 1 g; cholesterol: 4 mg; sodium: 328 mg; total fiber: 5 g; protein: 11 g; carbohydrate: 51 g; potassium: 436 mg

Green Beans Sauté

1 lb. fresh or frozen green beans, cut into 1-inch pieces
1 Tbsp. vegetable oil
1 large yellow onion, halved lengthwise, thinly sliced
1/2 tsp. salt
1/8 tsp. black pepper
1 Tbsp. fresh parsley, minced

If using fresh green beans, cook in boiling water for 10 to 12 minutes or steam for 2 to 3 minutes until barely fork tender. Drain well. If using frozen green beans, thaw first.

Heat oil in large skillet. Sauté onion until golden. Stir in green beans, salt, and pepper. Heat through. Before serving, toss with parsley.

Yield: 4 servings; serving size: 1/4 cup

Each serving provides: Calories: 64; total fat: 4 g; saturated fat: less than 1 g; cholesterol: 0 mg; sodium: 282 mg; total fiber: 3 g; protein: 2 g; carbohydrate: 8 g; potassium: 161 mg

Italian Vegetable Bake

1 28-oz. can whole tomatoes
1 medium onion, sliced
1/2 lb. fresh green beans, sliced
1/2 lb. fresh okra, cut into 1/2-inch pieces (or 1/2 of 10-oz. package frozen, cut)
3/4 c. green pepper, finely chopped
2 Tbsp. lemon juice
1 Tbsp. fresh basil, chopped, or 1 tsp. dried basil, crushed
1 1/2 tsp. fresh oregano leaves, chopped, or 1/2 tsp. dried oregano, crushed
3 medium zucchini, cut into 1-inch cubes
1 medium eggplant, pared, cut into 1-inch cubes
2 Tbsp. Parmesan cheese, grated

Drain and coarsely chop tomatoes. Save liquid. Mix together tomatoes, reserved liquid, onion, green beans, okra, green pepper, lemon juice, and herbs. Cover and bake at 325˚ F for 15 minutes.

Mix in zucchini and eggplant. Continue baking, covered, 60 to 70 minutes more or until vegetables are tender. Stir occasionally.

Just before serving, sprinkle top with Parmesan cheese.

Yield: 18 servings; serving size: 1/2 cup

Each serving provides: Calories: 27; total fat: less than 1 g; saturated fat: less than 1 g; cholesterol: 1 mg; sodium: 86 mg; total fiber: 2 g; protein: 2 g; carbohydrate: 5 g; potassium: 244 mg

Smothered Greens

3 c. water

1/4 lb. smoked turkey breast, skinless

1 Tbsp. fresh hot pepper, chopped

1/4 tsp. cayenne pepper

1/4 tsp. cloves, ground

2 cloves garlic, crushed

1/2 tsp. thyme

1 scallion, chopped

1 tsp. ginger, ground

1/4 c. onion, chopped

2 lb. greens (mustard, turnip, collard, kale, or mixture)

Place all ingredients except greens into large saucepan and bring to boil. Prepare greens by washing thoroughly and removing stems. Tear or slice leaves into bite-size pieces. Add greens to turkey stock. Cook for 20 to 30 minutes until tender.

Yield: 5 servings; serving size: 1 cup

Each serving provides: Calories: 80; total fat: 2 g; saturated fat: less than 1 g; cholesterol: 16 mg; sodium: 378 mg; total fiber: 4 g; protein: 9 g; carbohydrate: 9 g; potassium: 472 mg

Vegetable Stew

3 c. water

1 cube vegetable bouillon, low sodium

2 c. white potatoes, cut into 2-inch strips

2 c. carrots, sliced

4 c. summer squash, cut into 1-inch squares

1 c. summer squash, cut into 4 chunks

1 15-oz. can sweet corn, rinsed, drained (or 2 ears fresh corn—1 1/2 c.)

1 tsp. thyme

2 cloves garlic, minced

1 scallion, chopped

1/2 small hot pepper, chopped

1 c. onion, coarsely chopped

1 c. tomatoes, diced

Add other favorite vegetables, such as broccoli and cauliflower

Put water and bouillon in large pot and bring to a boil. Add potatoes and carrots, simmer for 5 minutes. Add remaining ingredients, except for tomatoes, and continue cooking for 15 minutes over medium heat.

Remove 4 chunks of squash and puree in blender. Return pureed mixture to pot and cook for 10 minutes more. Add tomatoes and cook for another 5 minutes.

Remove from flame and let sit for 10 minutes to allow stew to thicken.

Yield: 8 servings; serving size: 1 1/4 cups

Each serving provides: Calories: 119; total fat: 1 g; saturated fat: less than 1 g; cholesterol: 0 mg; sodium: 196 mg; total fiber: 4 g; protein: 4 g; carbohydrate: 27 g; potassium: 524 mg

New Potato Salad

16 (5 c.) small new potatoes
2 Tbsp. olive oil
1/4 c. green onions, chopped
1/4 tsp. black pepper
1 tsp. dill weed, dried

Thoroughly clean potatoes with vegetable brush and water. Boil potatoes for 20 minutes or until tender. Drain and cool potatoes for 20 minutes.

Cut potatoes into fourths and mix with olive oil, onions, and spices. Refrigerate and serve.

Yield: 5 servings: serving size: 1 cup

Each serving provides: Calories: 187; total fat: 6 g; saturated fat: 1 g; cholesterol: 0 mg; sodium: 12 mg; total fiber: 3 g; protein: 3 g; carbohydrate: 32 g; potassium: 547 mg

Apricot-Orange Bread

1 6-oz. package dried apricots, chopped
2 c. water
2 Tbsp. margarine
1 c. sugar
1 egg, slightly beaten
1 Tbsp. orange peel, freshly grated
3 1/2 c. all-purpose flour, sifted
1/2 c. fat-free dry milk powder
2 tsp. baking powder
1 tsp. baking soda
1 tsp. salt
1/2 c. orange juice
1/2 c. pecans, chopped

Preheat oven to 350° F. Lightly oil two 9- by 5-inch loaf pans. Cook apricots in water in covered medium-size saucepan for 10 to 15 minutes or until tender but not mushy. Drain and reserve 3/4 cup liquid. Set apricots aside to cool.

Cream together margarine and sugar. By hand, beat in egg and orange peel. Sift together flour, dry milk, baking powder, soda, and salt. Add to creamed mixture alternately with reserved apricot liquid and orange juice. Stir apricot pieces and pecans into batter.

Turn batter into prepared pans. Bake for 40 to 45 minutes or until bread springs back when lightly touched in center.

Cool for 5 minutes in pans. Remove from pans and completely cool on wire rack before slicing.

Yield: 2 loaves; serving size: 1/2-inch slice

Each serving provides: Calories: 97; total fat: 2 g; saturated fat: less than 1 g; cholesterol: 6 mg; sodium: 113 mg; total fiber: 1 g; protein: 2 g; carbohydrate: 18 g; potassium: 110 mg

Homestyle Biscuits

2 c. flour

2 tsp. baking powder

1/4 tsp. baking soda

1/4 tsp. salt

2 Tbsp. sugar

2/3 c. 1% fat buttermilk

3 1/3 Tbsp. vegetable oil

Preheat oven to 450° F. In medium bowl, combine flour, baking powder, baking soda, salt, and sugar. In small bowl, stir together buttermilk and oil. Pour over flour mixture and stir until well mixed.

On lightly floured surface, knead dough gently for 10 to 12 strokes. Roll or pat dough to 3/4-inch thickness. Cut with 2-inch biscuit or cookie cutter, dipping cutter in flour between cuts. Transfer biscuits to an ungreased baking sheet.

Bake for 12 minutes or until golden brown. Serve warm.

Yield: 15 servings; serving size: 1 2-inch biscuit

Each serving provides: Calories: 99; total fat: 3 g; saturated fat: less than 1 g; cholesterol: less than 1 mg; sodium: 72 mg; total fiber: 1 g; protein: 2 g; carbohydrate: 15 g; potassium: 102 mg

Rainbow Fruit Salad

For fruit salad

1 large mango, peeled, diced

2 c. fresh blueberries

2 bananas, sliced

2 c. fresh strawberries, halved

2 c. seedless grapes

2 nectarines, unpeeled, sliced

1 kiwi fruit, peeled, sliced

For honey-orange sauce

1/3 c. unsweetened orange juice

2 Tbsp. lemon juice

1 1/2 Tbsp. honey

1/4 tsp. ground ginger

dash nutmeg

Prepare the fruit. Combine all ingredients for sauce and mix. Just before serving, pour honey-orange sauce over fruit.

Yield: 12 servings; serving size: 4-oz. cup

Each serving provides: Calories: 96; total fat: 1 g; saturated fat: less than 1 g; cholesterol: 0 mg; sodium: 4 mg; total fiber: 3 g; protein: 1 g; carbohydrate: 24 g; potassium: 302 mg

1-2-3 Peach Cobbler

1/2 tsp. ground cinnamon

1 Tbsp. vanilla extract

2 Tbsp. cornstarch

1 c. peach nectar

1/4 c. pineapple juice or peach juice (if desired, use juice reserved from canned peaches)

2 16-oz. cans peaches, packed in juice, drained (or 1 3/4 lb. fresh), sliced

1 Tbsp. tub margarine

1 c. dry pancake mix

2/3 c. all-purpose flour

1/2 c. sugar

2/3 c. evaporated skim milk

1/2 tsp. nutmeg

1 Tbsp. brown sugar

nonstick cooking spray

Combine cinnamon, vanilla, cornstarch, peach nectar, and pineapple or peach juice in saucepan over medium heat. Stir constantly until mixture thickens and bubbles. Add sliced peaches to mixture. Reduce heat and simmer for 5 to 10 minutes.

In another saucepan, melt margarine and set aside. Lightly spray 8-inch square glass dish with cooking spray. Pour hot peach mixture into dish.

In a bowl, combine pancake mix, flour, sugar, and melted margarine. Stir in milk. Quickly spoon this over peach mixture. Combine nutmeg and brown sugar. Sprinkle on top of batter.

Bake at 400° F for 15 to 20 minutes or until golden brown. Cool and cut into 8 pieces.

Yield: 8 servings: serving size: 1 piece

Each serving provides: Calories: 271; total fat: 4 g; saturated fat: less than 1 g; cholesterol: less than 1 mg; sodium: 263 mg; total fiber: 2 g; protein: 4 g; carbohydrate: 54 g; potassium: 284 mg

Summer Breezes Smoothie

1 c. fat-free plain yogurt

6 medium strawberries

1 c. pineapple, crushed, canned in juice

1 medium banana

1 tsp. vanilla extract

4 ice cubes

Place all ingredients in blender and puree until smooth. Serve in frosted glass.

Yield: 3 servings; serving size: 1 cup

Each serving provides: Calories: 121; total fat: less than 1 g; saturated fat: less than 1 g; cholesterol: 1 mg; sodium: 64 mg; total fiber: 2 g; protein: 6 g; carbohydrate: 24 g; potassium: 483 mg

GLOSSARY

adventitia—Outer layer of the arterial wall.

aerobic fitness—Also called cardiovascular fitness, aerobic fitness refers to the body's capacity, especially the heart and cardiovascular system, to exercise. Aerobic means exercising when adequate oxygen is being delivered to all tissues. Activities in this class of exercise include walking, jogging, and cycling.

amino acids—Group of nitrogenous organic compounds that serve as the structural units of proteins and are essential to human metabolism.

anaerobic fitness—Refers to muscular fitness and the skeletal muscles' ability to do work, or their strength and endurance. Anaerobic means exercising in the absence of oxygen; in other words, oxygen does not need to be available for the exercising to be completed. Activities usually last less than a minute and include weightlifting or exercises requiring large amounts of work in short time periods.

aorta—Largest artery in the body. It supplies blood to all of the body, and it begins in the left ventricle of the heart.

arteriosclerosis—Group of cardiovascular disorders causing artery walls to thicken and harden.

atherosclerosis—Form of arteriosclerosis associated with lipid and plaque formation on the inner lining of the arteries.

bad cholesterol (LDL-C)—Involved in the movement of cholesterol from the digestive-absorption process. LDL-C becomes "bad" when found in excessive amounts in the blood (more than 100 mg/dL).

bile-acid sequestrants—Lipid-lowering medication that reduces the amount of cholesterol absorbed from intestinal bile acids.

calorie—Unit of energy used to define the energy value of foods (also see kilocalorie).

carbohydrate—Molecules that include starches, fiber, and simple sugars. Carbohydrate is found largely in bread-type foods such as cereal, vegetables, and pasta.

cardiovascular fitness—See aerobic fitness.

catheterization of the heart—Insertion of a catheter into an artery of the leg moved to the aorta and the heart. This allows pictures of the arteries to be taken showing plaque formation, blockages, and their location. This procedure is the primary method for diagnosing atherosclerosis.

cholesterol—Fat found in most animal tissues that is used to build cell membranes and structures and is a base component for steroid hormone synthesis. Excessive levels have been associated with increased risk for developing premature heart disease.

cholesterol-absorption inhibitors—New class of drugs designed to inhibit the absorption of dietary and biliary cholesterol across the intestinal wall.

complex carbohydrate—Starch, or foods containing not only carbohydrate but also fiber and other nutrients, providing the body with minerals, vitamins, and naturally occurring sugars.

concentric contraction—The portion of a muscle contraction where the muscle shortens.

coronary arteries—Arteries that supply blood to the heart. The primary arteries are the left and right coronary arteries that originate from the aorta. Other coronary arteries branch from these two main arteries and supply blood to the tissues of the heart.

coronary artery disease—Also called coronary heart disease or heart disease; refers to the narrowing of the arteries that supply blood to the heart. This narrowing is the result of inflammation and plaque formation that is composed of fats as well as other substances, including platelets, fibrin, calcium, and connective tissue.

creatine phosphokinase (CPK)—Enzyme found predominantly in the heart, brain, and skeletal muscles. When the blood CPK level is substantially elevated, it usually indicates injury or stress to one or more of these areas.

diabetes—The inability to transport glucose from the blood into cells. In type 1 (insulin-dependent) diabetes, the pancreas releases inadequate insulin. In type 2 (non-insulin-dependent) diabetes, absolute plasma insulin levels range from normal to high, but relatively low in relation to plasma glucose levels. Also called gradual-onset diabetes, type 2 diabetes usually occurs in obese people over the age of 35.

diverticulosis—Condition that causes pouch or sac openings to develop in the gut or bladder.

eccentric contraction—The portion of a muscle contraction where the muscle is lengthened.

endogenous fat—Fat produced by the liver. It is another source of VLDL, which becomes the main transport vehicle for triglycerides and is acted on by enzymes causing further release of FFAs. As VLDL breakdown continues, many smaller lipoprotein LDL particles are assembled.

endothelium—The cells lining the innermost layer, or intima, of arteries, veins, and the heart.

endurance exercise training—Exercise program that involves large muscle groups doing rhythmic movements and for more than several minutes. Also called aerobic or cardio training, the emphasis of this form of exercise is to develop the cardiovascular system's endurance. Examples include walking, running, swimming, rowing, stepping, biking, and dancing.

enzyme—Various organic substances produced in plant and animal cells that cause changes in other substances by promoting action.

exercise intensity—The work rate of exercise, or how hard you are working. Other descriptions of intensity include low, moderate, and high or vigorous exercise. Many exercise professionals use the terms *percentage of maximal functional capacity* or *percentage of maximal oxygen consumption*. Light intensity includes any activity more strenuous than sleeping and less strenuous than a brisk walk. Moderate intensity includes activities such as brisk walking that represent about 3 to 6 METs of work. When doing this kind of activity, you should be able to walk at a pace between three to four miles per hour. Vigorous intensity includes any activity that requires work greater than 6 METs. An example of this kind of activity is jogging or running at a pace greater than five miles per hour.

exogenous fat—Fat that is absorbed during digestion. Dietary fat is digested by the small intestine and absorbed as fatty acids and cholesterol. These absorbed lipids combine with apolipoproteins and are packaged into the center or core of large chylomicrons, which are released into the blood through the thoracic duct where they are free to move around the body.

familiar dysbetalipoproteinemia—An inherited disorder in which both cholesterol and triglycerides are elevated in the blood.

familial heterozygous hypercholesterolemia—An autosomal dominant disorder that causes severe elevations in total cholesterol and LDL-C.

fasting—Abstaining from eating for a period of time. In the measurement of blood lipids and lipoproteins and blood glucose, the normal standard fasting period is 8 to 14 hours. Water is allowed. Also referred to as the postabsorptive state.

fat—Greasy substance found in animal products and some plant products. Certain types of fat have greater association with chronic diseases like heart disease.

fat-soluble vitamins—Vitamins including A, D, E, and K that are stored in the liver and fatty tissues and are eliminated much more slowly than water-soluble vitamins. Because fat-soluble vitamins are stored for long periods, they generally pose a greater risk for toxicity when consumed in excess.

fibric acid derivatives—Drugs that are effective in lowering triglycerides and increasing HDL-C or "good" cholesterol. These medications can also somewhat reduce LDL-C or "bad" cholesterol.

fibrolipid plaque—Advanced form of plaque containing a lipid core covered with a connective-tissue fibrous covering or cap.

free fatty acids (FFAs)—Long-chain single linked carbon atoms referred to as a saturated fatty acid. This carbon chain contains no other unsaturated linkages (containing double bonds) between carbon atoms. A free fatty acid containing a carbon chain that possesses one or more double or triple bonds is an unsaturated fatty acid.

free radicals—Highly unstable, reactive oxygen molecules found in the blood. Oxidized LDL-C readily adheres to the endothelial arterial wall lining and is much more likely to form arterial plaque. Oxidized LDL can also cause other damage to the lipid membranes of the intimal and medial cells.

fructose—Simple sugar often found in fruits.

glucose—Simple sugar that makes up larger sugar molecules or is easily used for energy.

glucose intolerance—Group of diseases characterized by abnormally high fasting blood glucose (glucose that is measured after an individual has not eaten for 10 to 14 hours) and associated with diabetes. Fasting blood glucose values greater than 110 mg/dL mean the risk of developing diabetes in the next few years is great. Also called abnormal glucose tolerance.

good cholesterol (HDL-C)—Involved in the reverse cholesterol transport process. Excess cholesterol is removed from the peripheral circulation and moved by HDL to the liver where the cholesterol is removed from the HDL particle and excreted as bile into the small intestine.

hard plaque—Composed of fats, mostly cholesterol, but also triglycerides and phospholipids, as well as other substances including platelets, fibrin, calcium, and connective tissue.

heart attack—See myocardial infarction.

heart disease—See coronary artery disease.

homocysteine—An amino acid that, when found in excessive amounts in the blood, results in an increased risk of heart disease. This excess is brought on by either genetics or a deficiency in an enzyme called cystathionine synthase.

hydrogenated oils—Group of oils that are stabilized via hydrogen to provide a longer shelf life. These oils are a by-product of the process that creates trans-fatty acids, which can increase LDL-C levels.

hypercholesterolemia—Implies only elevated blood cholesterol levels.

hypertension—High blood pressure, which is defined as a systolic pressure of 140 mmHg and a diastolic pressure of 90 mmHg.

hypertriglyceridemia—Denotes only elevated blood triglyceride.

insoluble fiber—Indigestible fiber that helps remove toxins from the colon and promote regular bowel movements. Insoluble fiber is found in whole-wheat products, fruit skins, and green beans.

insulin—Hormone secreted by the pancreas. This peptide hormone promotes glucose utilization, protein synthesis, and the formation and storage of lipids.

insulin resistance—Develops when cells in the body are unable to respond to insulin's signals. This causes blood glucose levels to become elevated, and as a result, the pancreas produces even more insulin. Because the cell cannot respond to the insulin signals, blood glucose becomes excessively high. Elevated insulin resistance as well as elevated insulin levels change the way the body stores energy, causing the body to divert more energy into fat stores. This condition is associated with non-insulin-dependent diabetes.

intima—The innermost layer of the arterial wall; contains the endothelium.

isoflavone—Natural estrogen found in soy products that helps counteract endometriosis symptoms and menopausal symptoms and guard against osteoporosis.

kilocalorie—Energy unit of 1,000 calories used in defining the energy value of foods and energy expenditure. Also referred to as one large calorie or 1,000 calories.

LDL receptor pathway—Describes the process for the normal movement of cholesterol into cells.

lipemia—An abnormally high concentration of blood lipids.

lipids—Any of a group of organic compounds consisting of fats (e.g., cholesterol, triglycerides, phospholipids) and other substances of similar properties. They are insoluble in water but are soluble in fat solvents and alcohol and are greasy to the touch.

lipoprotein(a)—Also referred to as Lp(a), this is a unique subclass of LDL in that it contains the apolipoprotein(a), which is very similar to blood plasminogen in chemical composition. Because Lp(a) is chemically similar to plasminogen, it prevents plasminogen from breaking up blood clots as well as completing its physiologic roles. As a result, blood clotting is enhanced, which in turn amplifies the later stages of heart disease. Generally, blood Lp(a) levels greater than 20 to 25 mg/dL are associated with a greatly increased risk for developing premature heart disease.

lipoprotein lipase (LPL)—Enzyme associated with the arterial walls whose principal function is to remove the triglyceride portion from chylomicrons and VLDL particles.

lipoproteins—Particles made up of cholesterol, triglycerides, phospholipids, and proteins. Because lipids are not soluble, meaning they do not mix with water-based solutions like blood and other bodily fluids, proteins must combine with lipids into lipoproteins in order to move the lipids throughout the body. The four general lipoprotein classifications are chylomicron, very low-density lipoprotein (VLDL), low-density lipoprotein (LDL), and high-density lipoprotein (HDL).

lumen—Open space in the interior of a vessel such as an artery where blood flows.

macrophage—Large scavenger cell that originates as a monocyte and ingests dead tissue and other degenerated material.

maximal oxygen consumption—The greatest amount of oxygen that the body can use. Also used as an indicator of physical fitness, it is determined in part by genetics, is measured during maximal exercise, and increases after exercise training.

media—The arterial wall layer found between the intimal and adventitial layers. This layer contains most of the smooth muscle cells in the arterial wall.

MET—Stands for "metabolic equivalent" and is a measurement of work and the body's ability to consume oxygen. One MET is equal to the amount of oxygen consumed at rest (3.5 milliliters of oxygen per kilograms of body weight per minute). A person doing 3 METs of work is consuming three times the amount of oxygen consumed at rest.

mode of exercise—The type of exercise performed. For example, running and bicycling are different exercise modes. The benefits of one mode over another depend on your exercise goals and preference. The important thing is to pick a mode of exercise that you will do.

monocyte—Circulating blood cell that is one of the first inflammatory responses. These cells attach to the endothelial layer of the arterial wall and eventually move into the endothelium to the intima, where they begin to ingest dead and degenerated tissue.

monounsaturated fat—Fatty acids that contain one double or triple bond and are capable of absorbing hydrogens. These fats can absorb more hydrogens and store more energy and are considered healthy fats when consumed in small amounts.

muscular fitness—See anaerobic fitness.

myocardial infarction (heart attack)—When part of the coronary arteries are completely narrowed due to plaque formation and blood flow is not able to move to the heart, the areas not receiving blood die because without blood no oxygen is delivered. The larger the area affected by reduced blood flow, the larger the heart attack and the greater the necrosis.

necrosis—Death of one or more cells or a portion of tissue resulting from irreversible damage.

niacin—B vitamin found in milk, wheat germ, meat, and other foods. Niacin or nicotinic acid is extremely useful in patients with low HDL-C levels and is better than any of the other lipid-lowering agents in elevating blood HDL-C while also reducing LDL-C triglyceride levels.

nitric oxide—Colorless, free radical gas that is a naturally occurring vasodilator (widens the lumen of blood vessels) and is formed in tissue like the endothelium.

nonresponders—Individuals who have less than expected or little or no change in their exercise responses or adaptations. In the case of blood lipids and lipoprotein profile changes, these individuals have little or no response after exercise training.

obesity—Having a body mass index of greater than or equal to 30 kg/m^2. It is also referred to as an abnormal amount of fat in the subcutaneous areas.

omega-3 fatty acids—Found in fish oils, particularly in cold-water fish, these acids help reduce overall blood cholesterol and LDL-C levels.

one-repetition maximum (1RM)—Test used to measure the maximal amount of weight that a person can lift in one repetition. The test is begun by underestimating the weight that a person can successfully move. Small amounts of weight are added until the person cannot complete the movement.

phospholipid—A blood lipid similar to triglycerides that combines two free fatty acids and one phosphate into one molecule.

phytoestrogens—Chemical compounds that include isoflavones, which are estrogen-like compounds that occur naturally in many plants and fungi and are biologically active in humans and animals. Soy, particularly tofu and miso, and citrus fruits, wheat, licorice, alfalfa, fennel, and celery are rich sources of phytoestrogens.

plasminogen—Forerunner to the enzyme plasmin and responsible for the dissolving of blood clots.

platelets—Irregularly shaped disks in the blood associated with the process of blood clotting.

polyunsaturated fat—Like monounsaturated fat except these types of fat contain more than one double or triple carbon bond. These fats can absorb more hydrogens and store more energy and are considered healthy fat when consumed in small amounts.

postabsorptive period—Period after a time of fasting, usually 8 hours. Under these standardized conditions, blood fats, including triglyceride concentrations, are stable, as is blood glucose.

postprandial period—Period up to 14 hours after a meal. During this time blood fats that are absorbed through the digestive process steadily rise and then decline. Blood fat levels return to before-meal levels after 8 to 14 hours. Exaggerated or prolonged lipemia (abnormally long period for blood fat to return to normal levels) is associated with increased risk of heart disease.

protein—Molecules composed of up to 20 essential amino acids that are found in meat products, nut products, and eggs.

repetition (rep)—The number of times you lift a weight in each set.

resistance exercise training—See weight training.

responders—Individuals who respond or adapt to exercise in an expected way. Responders must have the proper genetic characteristics that allow them to have an expected exercise response. See also nonresponders.

reverse cholesterol transport—The transport of cholesterol by HDL from all parts of the cardiovascular system to the liver where it is broken down and excreted. Generally, blood HDL particles low in cholesterol and triglyceride content interact with other lipoproteins such as VLDL, IDL, and LDL and collect cholesterol and triglycerides. When the HDL is mature (can no longer collect other lipids), it returns to the liver where the cholesterol and triglycerides are removed and the HDL minus cholesterol and triglycerides is placed back into the circulation. Increased HDL-C levels means the risk of premature heart disease is reduced.

rhabdomyolysis—Condition when a muscle structure called the sarcolemma becomes damaged and the cells leak toxins and proteins into the bloodstream. Results from a direct injury to muscle fibers and can occur from statin use.

set—Group of successive exercises or repetitions performed without a rest period.

simple carbohydrate—Refined sugars (glucose) found in candy, table sugar, and syrup. These sugars are broken down by the body for quick energy.

soft plaque—Form of atherosclerosis found on the inner lining of arterial walls. This type of plaque is composed of fats, mostly cholesterol, some triglycerides, and phospholipids. To a much lesser degree other substances such as platelets, fibrin, calcium, and connective tissue are also found. Soft plaque is more susceptible to rupture than hard plaque.

soluble fiber—Digestible fiber that alters the digestion process while helping to lower LDL-C levels, decreasing the risk of heart disease. Sources of soluble fiber include oat bran, oranges, and carrots.

statin—a class of lipid-lowering medication also referred to as 3-hydroxy-3-methylglutaryl coenzymeA reductase inhibitors (HMG-CoA reductase inhibitors) that reduces the amount of cholesterol made in the liver.

thrombus—Blood clot found in the cardiovascular system that may or may not block the lumen and may attach to the vessel wall or plaque formation.

trans-fatty acids—Fat that comes from an industrial process that stabilizes polyunsaturated fat. This manufactured fat has the potential to cause cancer and heart disease.

triglycerides—A blood lipid that combines three free fatty acids into one molecule and has many functions including the storage of fat and the construction of cell membranes.

type III hyperlipidemia—Develops because of a defect in VLDL clearance. Individuals with this condition have difficulty removing triglyceride-rich VLDL particles from the blood, resulting in elevations of cholesterol and triglycerides. Also known as familiar dysbetalipoproteinemia.

weight training—Exercises that move body parts through a full range of motion with a weight or resistance. This type of exercise can only be sustained for brief time periods. The emphasis of this form of exercise training is the development of muscular strength and endurance.

REFERENCES

American College of Sports Medicine (ACSM). 2000. *ACSM's guidelines for exercise testing and prescription*. 6th ed. Baltimore: Lippincott Williams & Wilkins.

———. 2001. *ACSM's resource manual for guidelines for exercise testing and prescription*. 4th ed. Baltimore: Lippincott Williams & Wilkins.

———. 2005. *ACSM's guidelines for exercise testing and prescription*. 7th ed. Baltimore: Lippincott Williams & Wilkins.

American Heart Association (AHA). 2005. *Heart Disease and Stroke Statistics—2005 Update*. Dallas, Texas: American Heart Association.

Behall, K.M., D.J. Scholfield, and J. Hallfrisch. 1997. Effect of beta-glucan level in oat fiber extracts on blood lipids in men and women. *Journal of the American College of Nutrition* 16:46-51.

DeBusk, R.F., U. Stenestrand, M. Sheehan, and W.L. Haskell. 1990. Training effects of long versus short bouts of exercise in healthy subjects. *American Journal of Cardiology* 65(15):1010-3.

Donnelly, J.E., D.J. Jacobsen, K.S. Heelan, R. Seip, and S. Smith. 2000. The effects of 18 months of intermittent vs. continuous exercise on aerobic capacity, body weight and composition, and metabolic function in previously sedentary, moderately obese females. *International Journal of Obesity and Related Metabolic Disorders* 24:566-572.

Durstine, J.L., P.W. Grandjean, C.A. Cox, and P.D. Thompson. 2002. Lipids, lipoproteins, and exercise. *Journal of Cardiopulmonary Rehabilitation* 22:385-398.

Durstine, J.L., P.W. Grandjean, P.G. Davis, M.A. Ferguson, N.L. Alderson, and K.D. DuBose. 2001. Blood lipid and lipoprotein adaptations to exercise: A quantitative analysis. *Sports Medicine* 31(15):1033-62.

Durstine, J.L., M.D. Senn, B.P. Bartoli, P. Sparling, G.E. Wilson, and R.R. Pate. 1987. Lipid, lipoprotein and iron status of elite and good women runners. *International Journal of Sports Medicine* 8(supplement):119-123.

Durstine, J.L., and P.D. Thompson. 2001. Exercise in the treatment of lipid disorders. *Cardiology Clinics* 19(3):471-488.

Feigenbaum, M.S. 2001. Exercise prescription for healthy adults. In *Resistance Training for Health and Rehabilitation*, eds. J.E. Graves and B.A. Franklin, 107. Champaign, IL: Human Kinetics.

Grundy, S.M., J.I. Cleeman, C.N. Bairey Merz, H.B. Brewer, L.T. Clark, D.B. Hunninghake, R.C. Pasternak, S.C. Smith, N.J. Stone. 2004. Implications of recent clinical trials for the National Cholesterol Education Program Adult Treatment Panel III Guidelines. *Circulation* 110:227-239.

Gyntelberg, F., R. Brennan, J. Holloszy, G. Schonfeld, M. Rennie, and S.W. Weidman. 1977. Plasma triglyceride lowering by exercise despite increased food intake in patients with type-IV hyperlipoproteinemia. *American Journal of Clinical Nutrition* 30:716-720.

Halle, M., A. Berg, D. Konig, J. Keul, and M.W. Baumstark. 1997. Differences in the concentration and composition of low-density lipoprotein subfraction particles between sedentary and trained hypercholesterolemic men. *Metabolism* 46(2):186-91.

Hammer, W. 2003. That persistent muscle pain may be drug-induced. *Dynamic Chiropractic* 21(5).

Heber, D., I. Yip, J.M. Ashley, D.A. Elashoff, R.M. Elashoff, and V.L.W. Go. 1999. Cholesterol-lowering effects of a proprietary Chinese red yeast rice dietary supplement. *American Journal of Clinical Nutrition* 69:231-236.

Hu, F.B., J.E. Manson, and W.C. Willett. 2001. Types of dietary fat and risk of coronary heart disease: A critical review. *Journal of the American College of Nutrition* 20:5-19.

Kraus, W.E., J.A. Houmard, B.D. Duscha, K.J. Knetzger, M.B. Wharton, J.S. McCartney, C.W. Bales, S. Henes, G.P. Samsa, J.D. Otvos, K.R. Kulkarni, and C.A. Slentz. 2002. Effects of the amount and intensity of exercise on plasma lipoproteins. *New England Journal of Medicine* 347(19):1483-1492.

Morris, J., A. Kagan, D.C. Pattison, M. Gardnes, and P. Roffle. 1966. Incidence and prediction of ischemic heart disease in London busmen. *Lancet* ii:553-559.

National Cholesterol Education Program (NCEP). 1993. Expert Panel on Detection, Evaluation, and Treatment of High Blood Cholesterol in Adults (Adult Treatment Panel II). Second report of the National Cholesterol Education Program (NCEP). NIH Publication No. 93, 361, 662.

———. 2002. Expert Panel on Detection, Evaluation, and Treatment of High Blood Cholesterol in Adults (Adult Treatment Panel III). Third report of the National Cholesterol Education Program (NCEP). NIH Publication No. 02-5215.

Nicolosi, R., S.J. Bell, B.R. Bistrian, I. Greenberg, R.A. Forse, and G.L. Blackburn. 1999. Plasma lipid changes after supplementation with beta-glucan fiber from yeast. *American Journal of Clinical Nutrition* 70:208-212.

Poppitt, S.D. 2005. Postprandial lipaemia, haemostasis, inflammatory response and other emerging risk factors for cardiovascular disease: The influence of fatty meals. *Current Nutrition & Food Science* 1:23-34.

Ross, R., and J. Glomset. 1986. The pathogenesis of atherosclerosis. *New England Journal of Medicine: An Update* 314:496.

Sharma, R.D., T.C. Raghuram, and N.S. Rao. 1990. Effect of fenugreek seeds on blood glucose and serum lipids in type I diabetes. *European Journal of Clinical Nutrition* 44: 301-306.

Tjerk W., A. de Bruin, F.C. de Ruijter-Heijstek, D. Willem Erkelens, and A.P. van Beek. 1999. Menopause is associated with reduced protection from postprandial lipemia. *Arteriosclerosis, Thrombosis, and Vascular Biology* 19:2737.

U.S. Department of Health and Human Services (DHHS). 1996. Physical activity and health: A report of the surgeon general. Atlanta: CDC, NCCDPHP.

Willet, W.C., F. Sacks, A. Trichopoulou, G. Drescher, A. Ferro-Luzzi, E. Helsing, and D. Trichopoulos. 1995. Mediterranean diet pyramid: A cultural model for healthy eating. *American Journal of Clinical Nutrition* 61:1402S-1406S.

INDEX

Note: The italicized *f* and *t* following page numbers refer to figures and tables, respectively.

ABOUT THE AUTHOR

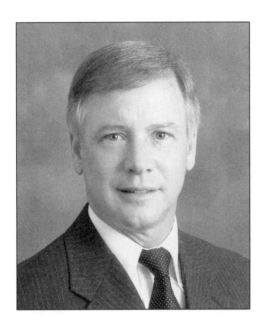

J. Larry Durstine, PhD, FACSM, is director of clinical exercise programs and a professor in the department of exercise science at the University of South Carolina. Since 1976 he has been involved in research focusing on the evaluation of exercise testing and training programs in both healthy people and those with chronic diseases and disabilities. Durstine has written more than 30 scientific publications regarding the impact of regular exercise on blood cholesterol. He also has written extensively on the subject of exercise testing and prescription and has served as editor for several American College of Sports Medicine (ACSM) books. Additionally, he is a fellow of ACSM and the American Association of Cardiovascular and Pulmonary Rehabilitation (AACVPR). Durstine was elected president of ACSM for the 2005-2006 term.

ABOUT ACSM

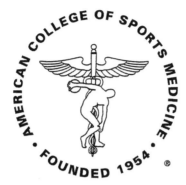

The **American College of Sports Medicine (ACSM)** is more than the world's leader in the scientific and medical aspects of sports and exercise; it is an association of people and professions exploring the use of medicine and exercise to make life healthier for all people.

Since 1954, ACSM has been committed to the promotion of physical activity and the diagnosis, treatment, and prevention of sport-related injuries. With more than 20,000 international, national, and regional chapter members in 80 countries, ACSM is internationally known as the leading source of state-of-the-art research and information on sports medicine and exercise science. Through ACSM, health and fitness professionals representing a variety of disciplines work to improve the quality of life for people around the world through health and fitness research, education, and advocacy.

A large part of ACSM's mission is devoted to public awareness and education about the positive aspects of physical activity for people of all ages from all walks of life. ACSM's physicians, researchers, and educators have created tools for the public, ranging in scope from starting an exercise program to avoiding or treating sport injuries.

ACSM's National Center is located in Indianapolis, Indiana, widely recognized as the amateur sports capital of the nation. To learn more about ACSM, visit www.acsm.org.

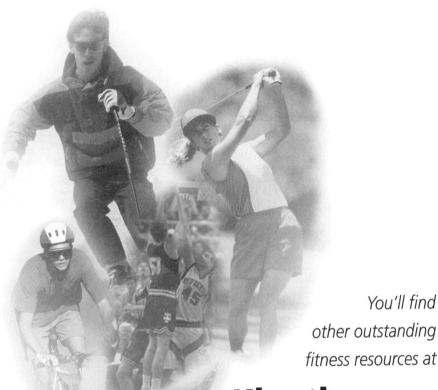